PLAYING THE PATHWAYS
OF MY BRAIN

PLAYING THE PATHWAYS
OF MY BRAIN

HOW A CONCERT PIANIST WITH MS ENJOYS PLEASURE
IN PERFORMANCE BY UNDERSTANDING HER MUSICAL BRAIN

OLGA BOBROVNIKOVA

authorHOUSE®

AuthorHouse™ UK Ltd.
1663 Liberty Drive
Bloomington, IN 47403   USA
www.authorhouse.co.uk
Phone: 0800.197.4150

Published by AuthorHouse   02/18/2014

ISBN: 978-1-4918-9266-4 (sc)
ISBN: 978-1-4918-9273-2 (e)

CONTENTS

LIST OF ILLUSTRATIONS

FOREWORD

F OR A CONCERT pianist to be diagnosed with Multiple Sclerosis is devastating, but Olga Bobrovnikova decided to fight her fate in two ways.

First she dedicated her talent to awareness and fundraising for MS and other neurological conditions.

Secondly she researched the neuroscience of music and the brain and has produced in this book, a fascinating blend of her life experience and a clear understanding of the neurological musical functions of her brain.

In the year originally intended as European Year of the Brain, and in the context the Bain Initiative of President Obama, this book is published with the intention of providing, musical knowledge for neurologists and neurological knowledge for musicians, also an interesting read for anyone who enjoys music.

For any performing musician she clearly argues a new, scientifically backed theory of performance based on the triangulation of physical, mental and emotional functions.

Using this "Triangle of Performance" can improve learning and practice and replace stage stress with enjoyment for the artist and the audience.

Read and reprogram your performance capability.

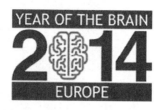

ACKNOWLEGEMENTS

D URING THE LAST two years, I often felt that my task was impossible, but with the help of many friends and several new acquaintances that I have yet to meet, I have reached the publishing line.

Firstly I have to thank my co-author and research partner Paul, for challenging the very foundations of music and also connecting the disparate pieces of science into new perceptions and ideas, initially inspired by the dedicated work of the Fondazione Mariani that promotes and publishes the work of the Neuromusic community.

Richard Muscat, Paul's Maltese friend for making us think about the idea of music and pleasure in the brain and his encouragement to keep going, as we struggled in early rewrites. My Mexican friend Jessica Verdi Tobon for her views on child development that fitted so well with the learning of music.

In the final stages I am indebted to those who took valuable time to read and comment particularly Cyril Hoschl for connecting me to Blanka Schaumann who was so encouraging and insistent that Larry Sherman should read the final draft.

I will be permanently indebted to Larry for his complimentary and critical comments and his corrections and contributions. I promised him that I would exonerate him from any responsibility for remaining crazy ideas. For these I blame Richard Lees for his words—"Outrageous comments are what is needed in a sea of ignorance."

For many others including; Sheila, Pennie, Mireille, Marina, Zdenka, Steven, Ken and Luc who all struggled through early drafts and their comments and suggestions kept us going.

The main thanks must go to Mary Baker who, when asked: where is music in the European brain project? simply replied "I think you had better do something".

So Mary and the European Brain Council, here it is— "Playing the Pathways of my brain" is for anyone, who like me either plays an instrument, loves music or is touched by any neurological condition.

Olga Bobrovnikova, GENVAL, January 2014

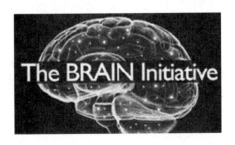

CHAPTER 1

Olga, multiple sclerosis (MS), and history

FORGIVE MY INDULGENCE in writing about myself, but I need to explain how piano performance changed for me when I was diagnosed with multiple sclerosis (MS). Before this, public recital was stressful, performance used to govern my life, but my MS diagnosis was the start of the path that led to each piano performance becoming a pleasure that I am able to share with the audience. The story of this journey from stress to pleasure is at the root of this book, which I have written in order to share my secrets with other performers.

For as long as I can remember I wanted to perform, and I once entertained ideas of being a ballet dancer or a singer. However, a decision, made when I was eight years old, meant that I would become a pianist, and from that moment I have loved playing the piano. Imagine at that young age the effect of the delivery of a grand piano to the twelfth floor of a Soviet block of flats; four strong men blocked the staircases for two hours as they manhandled the legless beast, disrupting the normal life of all of our neighbours, until finally my piano stood, with its legs reattached, virtually filling our lounge.

My parents were both university-graduated scientists, father working in missile defence and mother in computer management for energy distribution. In the West we would have been considered middle class, and in the Soviet Union our flat was better than average, a visible demonstration of our position in society. Our immediate neighbours were all of similar social status to my family, but a grand piano was clearly a special possession, and it was an important expression of my individuality.

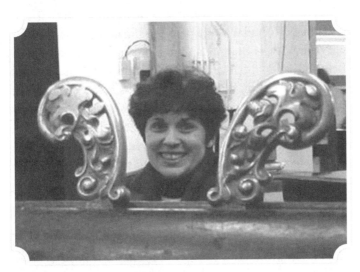

Olga's piano restoration

The piano was a pre-revolution Russian Schroeder, made in 1895; it was not a rebranded Red October piano from the confiscated factory. It was a special, shiny black beast from another time, with bulbous legs and elegant brass pedals and it dominated not only the living room of the flat where I lived, but my whole life. With it, I shared my love of the music from its own age: "Children's Album", "Swan Lake", "The Sleeping Beauty", "The Nutcracker", and "The Seasons", which I endlessly pestered my poor father to listen to, while he invented excuses to escape from endless repeats of "June" and "Waltz of the flowers"; Poor Father! Lucky Tchaikovsky?

My journey from private to public performance started in Moscow with my first piano teacher, Natalie Sherwood. It was she who advised my mother to buy the Schroeder that sits, forty years later, fully restored and reunited with me in my adopted Belgium home.

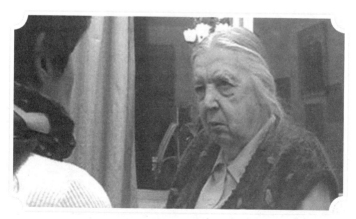

Olga and Natalie Sherwood

Natalie was born in 1925, the great-granddaughter of Vladimir Sherwood, architect of the National Historical Museum on Red Square. Her illustrious family with the English name were descendants of Joseph, the first Russian Sherwood, from Kent, who arrived in the country as a canal engineer, to work for Peter the Great (1672-1725). Natalie herself was a living link to the Russian Silver period; she was a student of Konstantin Igumnov (1873-1948), the Russian pianist, who knew Tchaikovsky and many other composers and artists who still inspire me today. She developed my instinctive love of music into emotional articulation that became the foundation of my performances.

The second big influence in my life was Musa Denisova at the Gnessin Junior School, who trained me with studies of Carl Czerny (1791-1857), as well as the precision of Johann Sebastian Bach (1685-1750), to establish my mental approach to performance.

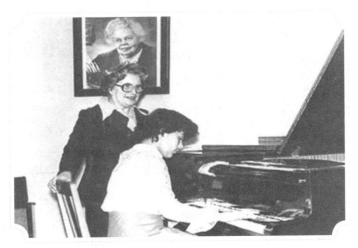

Olga, Musa Denisova, and Elena Gnessina

Another influence from this period was the book on Bach by Albert Schweitzer, first published in Russia in 1964, which my father bought for my fifteenth birthday. Rereading this recently, I realised that Schweitzer, a medical doctor and Nobel prize winner, identified and wrote about images and language in the music of Bach, but his views, which I now share, are not common among Bach specialists.

The picture of Musa and I was taken just before my graduation. I sit below a portrait of Elena Gnessina, one of the sisters that founded the Gnessin Musical School in 1895, the same year that my historic piano was built.

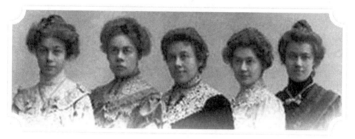

Gnessin sisters in the 1890s

At the Gnessin Junior School, my life was carefree and good, but it changed after the fateful decision to enter a degree course at the Moscow Conservatoire where I was accused of being too individualistic and was subjected to rigid rules, including the absolute rule of conformity.

When this senseless musical straitjacket was placed around Frédéric Chopin (1810-1849), it reduced me to confusion and to question the very meaning of music.

Fortunately, Natalie rescued me, and I survived and have the secret she gave me: I should always understand and believe what the music says.

Trying to discuss the meanings of Chopin led inevitably an emotional dialogue and then involvement with my professor, a famous concert pianist. The result was a scandalous affair and inevitable exposure; I was hauled in front of KOMSOMOL, the All-Union Leninist Young Communist League, tried, and "excommunicated". The ban prevented me from entering the high degree at the Moscow Conservatoire.

Soviet life was very uncomfortable for me even before this tragedy. On a student trip to Budapest in Hungary I was, like other classmates, "befriended" by the travelling security "minder". He made it clear that I would have no future as a pianist but a good career in security, if I was willing to submit to his attentions.

On another trip to an enforced agricultural camp, we intellectual students were forced to labour in the fields. I ended up with a severe fever and struggled to keep going. Shortly after, I collapsed in the Moscow Metro with paralysis of my legs and was hospitalised for weeks with what I was kindly told was a neurological infection. "Kind", because to have been told that I had multiple sclerosis at that time in Russia, would have ended all of my plans to become a pianist. I may have been confined to the flat as an invalid with mental problems.

However, after three months of hospitalisation and treatment, and having been rejected by the Moscow Conservatoire, I was lucky to get a postgraduate place back at the Gnessin Higher Musical Institute in Moscow to study for a masters degree in chamber music, thanks only to the efforts of my grandmother who intervened using her status as a "Hero of the War".

My illness highlighted my realisation that, in spite of the emotional engagement with music given to me by Natalie and the mental strength developed in me by Musa, I lacked the physical prowess to succeed in piano competitions and what they called the "academic music", which required strength, speed, and perfect accuracy, all so difficult as my hands are the size of an average ten-year-old, only just capable of spanning an octave. In addition, my "infection" had left me permanently fighting fatigue.

So practice and performance were a constant battle against my physical limitations, and a fear of the return of the neurological infection and temporary paralysis that could stop me playing at any time. Fortunately I did not discover I had MS for nearly 20 years, as I would probably have been unable to motivate myself in the knowledge that my neural system was incurably damaged with a very high chance of future degradation from increasing flares. Knowledge that the disease might take my memory, cognition and physical capability would probably have made me feel I was on a doomed path. How wrong I would have been, MS has changed my life, but in some strange way, the changes have been positive.

However, studying for the Gnessin high degree was quite different to studying at the Moscow Conservatoire, it was not simply a permanent round of learning, practice and criticism. My new curriculum included Chamber

Performance with Professor Valerie Samoliotov, Therapy for Music with Professor Vladimir Raikov and even a module on recording techniques.

The work on therapy was confusing, as the objective seemed to be to release the performer's inhibitions and allow his or her emotions to be free—quite the opposite of what was taught by the piano professors, who required total control and perfect adherence to the score.

In Chamber Music I set out with Marina Muravina, my piano partner, to prepare for international four-hands competitions. I was quite determined to get to France, the focus of my early academic education at School 48, one of the exclusive foreign language schools that usually led to service with the Foreign Office. I had grown up surrounded by translations of Western books, from Goethe to Mann, Shakespeare to Dickens, and Molière to Maupassant. I had been educated in French about France, and Paris was the destination of my dreams. So the International Chamber Music Competition was a reason to rehearse incessantly.

However, our application was turned down in spite of the recommendations of our professor, and I began to think that the offer of an alternative security career, may have been a missed opportunity, as my individualism was definitely going to make following a musical career very difficult and getting out of the Soviet Union virtually impossible.

But life is full of the unexpected, and when I went to a concert by violin virtuoso Mikhail Bezverkhny, I was captivated by his individuality. How come it is OK for violinists to be individuals, but it is not OK for pianists?

We talked, and then we played together; and ten weeks later, against the advice of members of my family and all of my friends, we were married in St Petersburg. A year later our son, Leon, was born.

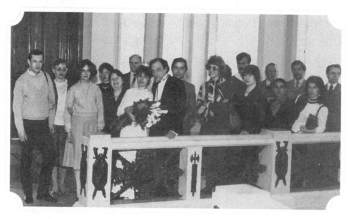

Olga's Wedding

Looking back, the wedding was a rather bizarre event and we never did identify one of the uninvited guests in the photograph who I recall, spoke to me in French!

One of Mikhail's biggest attractions for me was that he too wanted to get away. We planned to get to Israel and then to the USA, and an unexpected invitation gave us the opportunity to escape.

Mikhail had won several international competitions, including the Queen Elisabeth International Music Competition in Brussels, and he had been contacted by a Belgian impresario with the offer of a concert booking in Brussels.

Our most immediate problem was obtaining visas, not only for Mikhail and I but also our son. For years I had been subject to special rules because my father's work (in air defence) was classified as top secret. I believed that the chances of me getting permission to leave were slim, but with my son, almost zero. However, I had not realised that my father, who had been sick with Parkinson's disease (PD) and retired for more than two years at this point, was no longer considered to be a risk. Using his illness and the inability of my working mother to look after Leon, we applied for and got three exit visas.

We then had to secretly prepare to leave, discretely selling possessions for money, and illegally purchasing dollars for our trip. We nervously approached the scheduled day of departure, eventually arriving at the airport with two suitcases, two violins, and a viola. We were prevented from checking in because Leon was exactly two years old on the day of travel and therefore needed a ticket. The day before he could have travelled without a ticket, but now all of our plans were shattered. We stood feeling helpless, but then Mikhail realised that he had a hundred-dollar bill in his jeans. We bought a ticket for Leon, boarded the aeroplane, and flew to Belgium in February 1990 on a five-day visa with no intention of returning.

We planned a new life, one of two "individualist musicians" with their son and no money, but living free in the West, I also carried a brain full of rich musical memories . . .

CHAPTER 2

MS diagnosis and a book

THE STRESS OF Soviet restrictions was immediately replaced by the stress of adapting to Western freedom and a need to get work, find somewhere to live, and establish refugee status in a new and strange environment.

To my surprise I discovered that French was one of the languages of Belgium. So my education allowed me to adapt relatively quickly, and with the help of some very kind people we gained refugee status and permission to remain in Belgium. But hopes of onward travel to Israel or the USA were dashed as the United Nations (UN) convention required application for asylum to be made in the first country of arrival.

Finding musical bookings was not the most difficult thing; earning enough money to live on was the biggest challenge. Alongside being a mother and a housekeeper, I became not only a pianist but a part-time translator, a second-hand car exporter, and an agent for oligarchs en route to Cyprus.

Looking back, it is no wonder that my performances were erratic: Some were excellent, but some were far below the standard that Mikhail required. This state of affairs gradually destroyed our musical relationship and, finally, our marriage.

Six years after arriving in Belgium I found myself separated and a single mother, without support, having to build a new life again.

I took a part-time job as a buyer with a chain of CD shops, which as an independent artist in Belgium was the only economic way to pay compulsory health insurance and taxes. I began to rediscover my solo repertoire and give concerts, and in many ways this was a creative and happy period because my job required that I listen to all of the newly released CDs and browse the catalogues to make buying decisions.

It was like compact-disc heaven; all my spare time was spent listening to recordings, old and new, and I made some interesting discoveries and judgements regarding piano performances. I realised that the publicity of the CD distributors was only marginally worse than the opinions of the critics. By listening to hundreds of CDs, including several versions of the same work on occasions, it became evident that really great performances were very rare. There were a few good ones, but the majority were simply mechanical without any evident meaning. During ten years of working in the record retail industry, I realized that the taste and needs of the audience were out of step with the marketing objectives of the industry.

Even before the downloading era contributed to the collapse of the record industry, I was selling more old re-releases than the new, heavily marketed ones. This was not because of the price difference but simply because of customer preference, although admittedly I was involved in finding and offering these older recordings.

After one of my concerts a gentleman came up to me and asked for an autograph, and without going into detail regarding the next two years of indecision, you should know that I married him, and Leon and I became part of a reconstituted family. For the first time I enjoyed a normal life in the West: While I regularly played concerts and taught, I went on Club Med holidays, skiing, horse riding and weekend trips to the sea coast.

This ideal life, however, was suddenly shattered. For the first time in my life I had to cancel a concert. I found that I was unable to rehearse; my hands didn't respond, and the worst fears that I had carried with me since my spell in the Neurological Institute in Moscow were realised: I was diagnosed with multiple sclerosis. Immediately, visions of the tragedy of Jacqueline Du Pré, a classmate of my ex-husband Mikhail, overtook me as well as my new husband, who suffered a breakdown and tragically took his own life, being unable to face my challenging and possibly tragic future.

These events marked the end of a second life and the beginning of another, but thanks to my neurologist, who by proving that cortisone treatment was inappropriate for me, found a way to get interferon treatment reimbursed by the complex Belgian Healthcare system. So two years before the European treatment guidelines were published I was "privileged" to be on weekly interferon treatments. Now, twelve treatment years later, I am able to tell the story of how my MS prompted a search for the secrets of performance and the hidden emotional codes of music.

My diagnosis made me realise that MS affects the very parts of my brain and spinal cord needed for performance: it could cause the loss of myelin and thus the loss of high speed nerve cell impulses; the loss of synapses that form the circuits that allow me to move, sense, feel etc. and even the loss of nerve cells (neurons) themselves[1]. These changes could take my cognition, memory, coordination, or touché, at any time.

This forced me to think about a life without concerts. Pondering this awful possibility, I started to plan alternatives to piano performance, expanding my teaching, researching, and writing about the performers of the Silver Period. This led to my discovery of a piano work that was so challenging that I became obsessed with conquering it, simply to prove that there was nothing wrong with me. In fact at this lowest point of my life, alone and facing the inevitable decline of a life with MS, I found not one but two Pauls.

The challenging paraphrase for piano of the themes of the opera "Eugene Onegin" was written in the style and tradition of Liszt by a pianist called Paul Pabst, described on the CD sleeve as being a professor of the Moscow Conservatoire. In fact I didn't discover the track myself; it was brought to my attention by a very old mysterious gentleman who asked me to play the track for him.

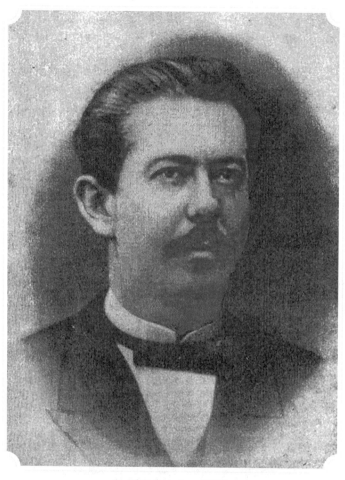

Paul Pabst circa 1878

As a graduate of the Moscow Conservatoire, I was confused about why I had never heard of Paul Pabst, the composer of this ultimate piano work. This made me research his story, and I was fascinated to discover that he was the teacher of Maria Gnessina, the founder of my first piano school, and that he also taught Igumnov, Natalie Sherwood's professor.

I discovered that he preferred to play a Schroeder piano, just like mine, and that he, like me, had been denigrated and rejected by the Moscow Conservatoire.

Paul number two was a customer in the CD shop who kindly asked what he could do to help, when he heard my tragic and distressing news. This Paul is still with me, a partner in research, music and life and . . . the co-author of this book. A strange echo from history seemed to confirm this relationship when I learned that Paul Pabst was married to an Olga whose Russianized name was Alexandra Petrovna.

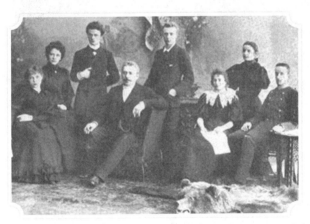

Paul Pabst and students—1895 (Igumnov extreme right)

Our research into Pabst and how he was lost from history allowed me to understand the historical changes that had taken place in piano performance over the last hundred years and the reason why I was so heavily criticised at the Moscow Conservatoire for excessive movement and individualism. My involvement with Pabst became almost obsessive but a very good way to ignore or fight MS.

This lost German-French soul and kindred spirit, who gave nineteen years of his life to Russian music, being decorated three times by the Tzar, became the subject of five years of research. The fascinating facts I uncovered, resulted in my writing historical novel that was published in Moscow, in Russian, under the title of (translated to English) *The Diaries of Alexandra Petrovna* or *A Paraphrase on a Sad Theme,* about the life of Pabst, his wife, their friend Tchaikovsky, and all of my heroes of the Silver Period. The proceeds of this book, now sadly out of print, were given to the All Russian MS Patient Organisation.

I also collected scores and recorded Pabst's other paraphrases of Tchaikovsky ballets and operas, his lost piano concerto, and the wonderful trio that he wrote in memory of his lifelong friend Anton Rubinstein.

I became so involved in the story of Pabst and his wife because I felt that I had been drawn into history, in order to resurrect his memory, and in Moscow in 2003, when I listened to the original Edison recordings from 1895 of Pabst playing Chopin and Schumann as well as his own works, I understood why his place in history needed to be restored. His performance was, in the words of Tchaikovsky, "of a pianist blessed by God". In the words of Von Meck to Tchaikovsky in 1880, Pabst was "*Le plus ultra*"[2].

This Paul Pabst, whose epitaph read, "Honoured Artist, Indefatigable Professor, Hardly simply a man", is definitely "*le plus ultra*", and the Edison wax cylinders of his performance in 1895 that I heard in Moscow and that have now been transferred to CD[3] are the crowning jewels of historic recordings of piano performances.

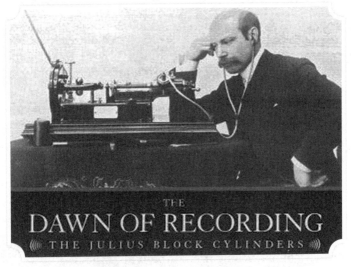

Marston Records—*The Dawn of Recording*

The music transcribed from these nearly inaudible wax cylinders, has given me all the evidence I need to understand just how much piano performance has changed in the past century. It has also given me confidence that my performance style, with its emotion and individualism, is historically valid, part of the real style of the Romantic era (c. 1850-1920).

I recommend that you listen to Pabst. You should ignore the century of noise—in both senses (audio and cultural). His unique fluid confidence, and jazz-like interpretations of Schumann and Chopin, reveal what music really is: a means of generating pleasure in our brains.

About the time I found Pabst, I read Norman Lebrecht's book *When the Music Stops . . . : Managers, Maestros and the Corporate Murder of Classical Music*,[4] and his analysis of the destruction of classical music by corporate greed and corruption, confirmed my understanding that only the notes of classical piano remain—the music has been almost completely lost.

I was convinced to argue for restoration of this "Old Style", but I needed to understand and objectively describe the art of performance, in order to identify precisely what had changed. What have we lost that previously created such empathy between pianists and their audience? In 2006 I wrote a small book called *Triangle of Performance* that suggested instinctive answers to the questions, but without any evidence to support my contentions.

But the most important effect of Pabst arriving in my life happened in 2003 in Malta, when I played a concert of his music that I had recently released on CD[5]. I was also at this time trying to persuade the director of the Maltese national orchestra to perform a Pabst piano concerto, written to celebrate the coronation of Tzar Alexander III and ignored for 120 years. I failed to get a performance in Malta, eventually succeeding in Moscow.

On the weekend of my Malta recital, the Annual Conference of the European MS Platform (EMSP) was taking place, and I made an invitation to the delegates to come to my concert to hear a pianist with MS. As my recital conflicted with their gala dinner, I arranged a special lunchtime concert for them in the Radisson Hotel, and that changed the focus of my life.

Since that moment, my performances have become increasingly involved in supporting multiple sclerosis awareness and fundraising, particularly in 2007, the twentieth anniversary year of the death of Jacqueline Du Pré from multiple sclerosis, when I gave twenty concerts in the UK, Europe, and New Zealand.

These activities for MS and other neurological conditions have gradually led to my interest in "Neuro Music", a branch of science that I hoped would answer some of the complicated questions about performance: How does my brain perform music? How do the brains of members of the audience respond?

This new book describes my two-year search through the published papers about music and neurology, to piece together how a performer's brain blends physical, mental, and emotional functions in order to create music.

One profound idea has guided me through the very complex texts regarding science and musicology; I believe that music is a means of communication, a language with simple objectives: to convey meaning and feelings to give pleasure.

Everything we understand is ultimately reduced to our own judgements of good/bad, like/dislike, need/don't need, fear/desire, and so forth, and these emotional values are stored with our memories. More simply put, we both understand and make decisions based on our memory of previous events, of which the oldest and most emotionally charged dominate our actions.

I believe that the language of music can, without words, directly address our memory and feelings; As performers we need to understand this and how we can use our own memory in order to transmit feelings with music, that will in turn access the memory and emotions of the audience.

If we do not do so, then we are in danger of delivering a aimless stream of notes and this I am sure was not the style of the romantic period.

CHAPTER 3

Performance and pleasure

P AUL PABST, THE lost pianist that I accidentally found, has allowed me to make up my own mind about the style of historic performance because of a musical miracle. Some Edison rolls have survived since 1892 through two world wars, the Russian Revolution, the Soviet era and 120 years of cultural destruction.

For legendary pianists like Chopin, Liszt, Clara Wike, Anton Rubinstein, Nikolai Rubinstein, and Hans von Bülow, we simply have written memories of how popular and exciting their concerts were.

For later superstars, such as Arthur Rubinstein, Vladimir Horowitz, Paderewski, Igumnov, Goldenweiser, and Rachmaninoff, we have recordings to judge their talents. What we hear is mixed; some are simply wonderful recordings, but many are "made for money" in the studio, without enjoyment, under the immense pressure of the need for perfection.

In fact we might have had an Edison recording of Anton Rubinstein if he had not refused on the grounds that he had no desire to make a permanent record of his mistakes[6].

One may play all the "Waltzes" of Chopin at one sitting, without a false note, or play the "Minute Waltz" in fifty-nine seconds, but is there meaning or pleasure for the performer or the audience?

When I listened to Pabst's rendering of the "Minute Waltz" ("Waltz in D-flat Major, Op. 64, No. 1"), which takes nearly two minutes, it is obvious that both pianist and audience are having fun and that Pabst incidentally, added extra notes and decoration, simply for pleasure.

Another great performer in my lifetime was Freddie Mercury of the group Queen, a gigantic superstar, who said about the audience: "It's my job to win them over, to make them feel they've had a good time."[7] I don't think that he realised that having a good musical time involves maximum neural pleasure.[8]

How many pianists believe this quotation? It appears so inappropriate for classical piano, but it isn't. Each type of performance—dance, music, and theatre—has the same objective: to entertain and provide pleasure.

Freddie, a pop idol, was also a lover of ballet and opera, successfully dancing with The Royal Ballet and topping global pop charts with opera diva Montserrat Caballé, his outstanding performance skill across all his activities was the ability to engage his audience and transmit his enjoyment.

Public performance is challenging for all musicians, but for those with neurological damage, it can be traumatic. By understanding more about my brain's musical processes, I have learned to reduce my stage fears and have discovered how to enjoy myself when I perform. The lessons I have learnt will be useful for anyone who performs in public and who wishes to enhance his or her confidence and reduce stress. But the starting point for any discussion must be: What is the purpose of musical performance?

I realised after suffering from neurological problems for a number of years, that in order to continue performing I needed to find pleasure for myself and that this would automatically lead to pleasure for the audience as we "engaged".

The realisation that my frail brain was the engine of my musical ability and the generator of my pleasure, made me think about the very nature of performance, and my first little book, which I subtitled, "Playing with the Mirror Neurons", was an attempt to explain how any performance can be effective, if physical, mental, and emotional functions are balanced.

The book was inspired by a friend who asked me a number of questions about music and performance. I remember becoming somewhat defensive, as I had difficulty answering apparently simple questions like: "Can one teach performance?" My instinctive answer was to say no, because I believed that the talent of musical icons like Arthur Rubinstein and Emil Gilles was "God given". The next question was: "What were you taught about performance?" Quite frankly, having graduated from the

Moscow Conservatoire and having obtained a high degree from the Gnessin Institute, I had to say that, I could only remember vague, negative, stylistic criticism, such as, "Don't slouch; sit up straight", "Don't move so much", "Don't vary the strict rhythm", and "We don't play Mozart like that", along with terminal trouble for being "too individualistic", the most serious crime in the Soviet music education system.

On reflection, I do remember two small things I was taught at the age of eight by Natalie Sherwood. Natalie would tell me to play like "sheep walking through the grass", to describe the gentle movements of legato slurs, and also said to me, "Don't jump—go smoothly over the bridge," to describe how to move between the keys.

My inquisitor also asked: "Why do some performances give pleasure and others are simply boring, when all the notes are played accurately?" He had just met, in the passenger lounge of Milan Airport, Professor Richard Muscat,[9] an expert on the neuroscience of pleasure, and they had discussed pleasure in the brain.

I was now trapped and interested to try to explain what makes a performance pleasurable. To do this I needed to explain why audiences so often differ in their judgement from critics, juries, and "academic musicians". I had to understand what motivates pianists, well past their physical best, to be willing to play for big audiences, knowing that they may play false notes.

Pop audiences go to see the artist; classical audiences, however, often go to hear the music, the artist being secondary. However, there are some classical musicians that attract audiences regardless of the music programme; why are they special?

I remember queuing all night long in 1986 for the comeback-concert of eighty-two-year-old Vladimir Horowitz in Moscow. His performance that night was so full of emotion, laughter, and tears that no one in the audience will ever forget the occasion or remember the wrong notes. This musical magician came from another time, the roots of his education were in the pre-radio era, the Russian Silver Period that I have studied for most of my life.

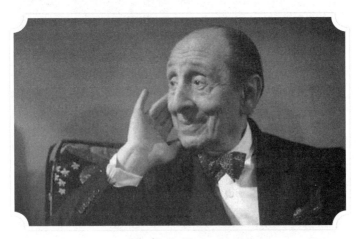

Vladimir Horowitz

Why did the audiences of Vladimir Horowitz or of the eighty-nine-year-old Arthur Rubinstein have unforgettable experiences at their legendary comeback events?

In particular, Horowitz, it seems, after many stressful performing years and a twenty-year break, finally discovered the secret of performance after the age of eighty.

It appears that Arthur Rubinstein always understood this secret, as can be read in his obituary in *The New York Times* that recalled him saying:

> "At every concert I leave a lot to the moment. I must have the unexpected, the unforeseen. I want to risk, to dare. I want to be surprised by what comes out. I want to enjoy it more than the audience. That way the music can bloom anew. It's like making love. The act is always the same, but each time it's different".[10]

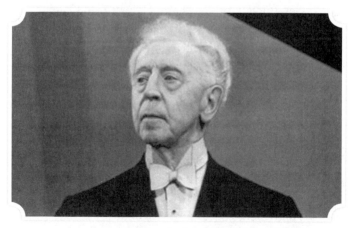

Arthur Rubinstein

Both of these iconic pianists played because they enjoyed performing, and they understood that the physical and mental effort has one objective: to engage the emotions of the audience.

This comes as no surprise because one of the simplest and earliest discoveries of neuro-music was that sex, drugs, and music stimulate the same pleasure centres in the brain.[11]

I started to read about music and the brain in order to explain the secrets of pleasure in music, but one of the first abstracts I read nearly made me give up. Forgive me for quoting it; I do so hoping that you may understand it. I still don't.

> "[T]he pianist decodes two types of information from the score in order to produce the desired piece of music. The spatial location of a note head determines which piano key to strike, and the various features of the note, such as the stem and flags determine the timing of each key stroke. We found that the medial occipital lobe, the superior temporal lobe, the rostral cingulate cortex, the putamen and the cerebellum process the melodic information, whereas the lateral occipital and the inferior temporal cortex, the left supramarginal gyrus, the left inferior and ventral frontal gyri, the caudate nucleus, and the cerebellum process the rhythmic information. Thus, we suggest a dissociate involvement of the dorsal visual stream in the spatial pitch processing and the ventral visual stream in temporal movement preparation."[12]

The only thing I take from this complex quotation is that the score is a problem. The quote explains to me why I can't play solo piano concerts when sight reading. Even when accompanying I prefer to have "the score in my head, not my head in the score".[13]

For me, a concert is about expressing ideas using the notes in my memory. It is like having a conversation in which I express my feelings, rather than reading a text.

This is contrary to the view of academic musicians who believe that a performance requires the perfect delivery of the notes from the score by following the notation in the most accurate and standard way possible.

While there is some pleasure and satisfaction to be gained by accurate delivery, this is small compared to the huge rush created by genuine empathy from the audience response.

I am confident in my instinctive understanding that performance is represented by a triangle[14] comprising three groups of functions:

- physical (body)
- mental (spirit).
- emotional (soul)

When these are balanced, the pianist's personality is revealed, an important step to empathy and sharing pleasure with the audience.

It is my observation that many great classical artists have unbalanced triangles, giving the impression of a hidden or flawed personality. It is not uncommon for performances to become so stressful and unrewarding that artists give up public performances, temporarily or permanently.

An example of this is Glen Gould who withdrew from public performance entirely, as did Horowitz himself for twenty years.

Having a perfectly balanced performance triangle is not enough on its own to engage an audience; we need to create a dialogue and establish a common mood.

I am in awe of the way that Freddie Mercury used to "warm up" his audiences, forcing them to copy his phrases and rhythms until they were sharing his arousal and mood.

Unfortunately, this is not appropriate to classical music where, typically, a pianist dressed like a penguin walks silently to the piano and, trance-like, ignores the audience before launching into a torrent of notes.

How different it is, when a few personal words are said and the choice of the introductory piece has a pace and tonality to entrain the audience with the artist.

But to delve deeper into the arts of performance, the balancing of triangles, and entrainment, we need to explain the processes of the brain and the attributes of music that contribute to performance and to audience pleasure.

CHAPTER 4

My broken brain

A FTER CANCELLING MY Christmas concert in 1999 I was referred to a neurologist, who in January 2000, told me that "I only had MS", meaning that it was not a tumour or brain cancer.

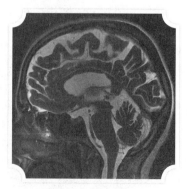

My brain MRI

But the diagnostic process and the first magnetic resonance imaging (MRI) of my brain was a very stressful event. To be injected with a chemical contrast agent, lie prone and immobile for 30 minutes and be slowly enveloped by a gigantic, noisy, magnetic monster, that recorded slices of image from the inside of my head and spine, was frightening. But the shock of the resulting picture immediately prompted a number of questions: Which symptom was caused by which lesion? Where will the next lesion appear? When would my fingers fail to respond? When will I forget my repertoire or be unable to read a score?

These questions that prompted me to try to find out more, were inspired by the elegance and beauty of the structure of the image of my brain, it was like a work of art. It was fascinating to wonder about the location of musical capability; just what does go on when I create a stream of notes? Why does it give me pleasure? How do I make the audience cry?

Seeking the answers to these questions, I have had an interesting, amazing, and often confusing journey, through more than a thousand scientific abstracts and articles on anatomy, neurology, history, and psychology.

The embryonic development of the brain is quite extraordinary, as the outer layer of the embryo grows into the neural tube, the top of this tube grows into our brain. I am indebted to Professor Larry S. Sherman, Ph.D. the Senior Scientist in the Division of Neuroscience at Oregon National Primate Research Center of Oregon Health and Science University for the full description below:

> ". . . . embryos, have structures that are flat
> sheets of cells called neuroectoderm. These

sheets fold (to form the "neural folds") and eventually form the neural tube. Cells divide within the walls of this tube. These cells are called neural stem cells. They will divide asymmetrically, giving rise to a new stem cell and a differentiated cell (either a neuron or some type of glial cell). One end of the tube divides much more than the other, forming the brain, while the rest of the tube will form the spinal cord. When we are born, we have far too many neurons (the electrical units of our brain that form the circuits of our nervous systems) and many die in the first years after birth. Furthermore, some of the axons of our neurons, along which electrical signals travel, become enveloped in myelin— an insulating substance that increases the speed of nerve impulses up to 100 times. The process of myelination continues into our twenties. In recent years, it has become clear that connections between neurons (synapses) can form throughout life and are important for learning and memory. Furthermore, we now know that we are capable making new neurons (a process called neurogenesis) throughout life, and that neurogenesis is also critical for learning and memory".

The first surprising fact is that, after developing in the womb the brain continues changing after birth until the age of twenty in response to usage, by forming and strengthening some connections while eliminating others.

The statement on the website of the American Society for Neuroscience[15] describes the process of myelination of the axons connecting one brain area to another as starting about the time of birth, moving from the back of the brain to the frontal lobes, which are responsible for judgement, insight, and impulse control and that this final myelination occurs as late as twenty or twenty-five years of age in the male.

I am also very happy, as a person with some brain damage, to learn that brain plasticity allows neural growth into old age, especially when assisted by fasting.[16]

So both the embryonic and post natal physical development of the brain seem to follow a quasi linear route, bottom to top and back to front.

This physical development is driven by functional needs derived from progressive use.

Just after Gipsy my dog died, I started to walk my neighbour's Alsatian puppy, and we followed the same route each day for several months. I was quite captivated by the changes that took place in the very young puppy, as the priority it would give to smell or hearing or sight gradually changed and finally became an integrated set, making an alert, fully functioning dog. The process seemed to be driven by need or wanting to do something and then by trial and error to achieve success. The achievements result in expecting more success by repeating the new tricks!

Do musicians learn in the same way, do their brains develop in any special way as they make music as well as listen and enjoy music?

Looking at the elegant structure of my brain MRI, I was inspired to discover more. Unfortunately, as I said, the more anatomy and physiology I read, the more confused I became.

My first simple understanding was that:
The bottom section of my brain, the part just above my spine, is concerned with automatic sensory functions associated with sleeping and arousal etc.

The middle section of the brain integrates the senses, is a communications centre, and the location of the pleasure-and-reward mechanisms.

The top section has two hemispheres of cortex, each with segments for making sense of the audio and visual and other sensory signals by reference to memory.

The front parts of the hemispheres are the most developed for emotional and strategic decisions and planning.

We have all observed new born babies and see how their visual skill develop in the first two weeks of life and I was not really surprised to discover a controversial theory that the physical capabilities and mental development of the newborn baby can be mapped to brain structures.

The theory goes:

As our brain contains a primeval element in the medulla, pons, mid-brain and four mammalian/human developments of the cortex, these "brain sections" are directly involved in the stages of post-natal development for mobility, visual, auditory, linguistic, tactile, and manual skills that are generally completed by five years of age. These include "three stages of response; reflex, vital and meaningful and four stages of understanding and expression; initial, early, primitive and sophisticated".[17]

These concepts of post-natal development indicate a structure for the musical processing functions of the brain based post-natal needs, where our instinctive detection and sensor functions connect to recognition and comprehension and learning functions that finally associate with our experiences in memory.

Each of these big functional processes is associated with reward and pleasure, (wanting, liking and anticipating) the basic mechanisms that drives the brain functions.[18]

For me as a musician, the concept is profound, as it indicates an essentially linear pathway for music through the hierarchy of our brain, which is partly instinctive, partly evolved, and partly socially derived using physical, mental, and emotional functions which all seemingly create pleasure.

My initial confusion, mainly based in ignorance, was also created by the complexity of anatomy and functionality that do not map in a simple way.

While we have a single reward mechanism it seems that evolution has reused it by creating several pathways to it. It also seems that mirror motor functions are well distributed and not simply a selection of mirror neurons. As far as music processing is concerned the mid-brain, it seems, is involved in all functions and it is evident that the same sound must be subject to both a sequence of linear and parallel processes which we enjoy as a single music experience.

It is not surprising that many researchers state that "the brain lights up like a Christmas tree when we listen to music".

So while there are no simple three-level functional structures, I think it is necessary to view the logical architecture as having three groups to help unravels the multitude of neural responses observed and studied by scientists.

CHAPTER 5

Pleasure from Parkinson's

M Y FATHER WAS diagnosed with Parkinson's disease (PD) at the age of thirty-nine, when I was just fifteen years old. As I watched his deterioration and his increasing dependence on Nakom medicine (Levodopa) the last thing I can remember is pleasure. It is therefore hard to imagine that some thirty years later I would be reading about the connections between Parkinson's and the reward systems in the brain that are also associated with human pleasure.

Remember it was my father's severe illness that finally removed his security status and allowed me to get an exit visa from the Soviet Union. It also allowed him to make one visit to Belgium, in 1991.

I never saw him again because shortly after returning to Moscow he entered a nursing home and one afternoon, following a visit from my mother, he, feeling better simply walked out of the door like Tolstoy, and disappeared. As his journey took him outside of the Moscow city area, so it was more than a year before we discovered what had happened.

It seems that he took a bus to the countryside and became disorientated and lost; we simply know that he was found dead and buried.

In 2004 I visited his snow-covered grave, in the middle of a birch wood, almost like a scene from "Snowstorm" the Alexander Pushkin novel.

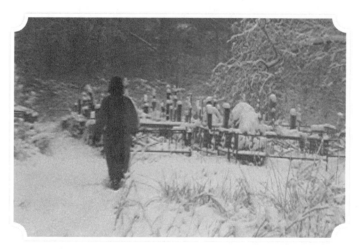

Olga visiting father's grave

So while my memories of Parkinson's are very sad, I was fascinated to read the research regarding three separate reward circuits (limbic, motor, and associative) that are damaged by the disease. These circuits all involve basal ganglia and dopamine reward.[19]

The brain chemistry and anatomy involved are still the subject of research, but the concept of three circuits that both excite and inhibit our responses, is generally accepted.

From this work I can imagine a complicated reward system for music that excites and inhibits, providing positive and negative rewards via three different circuits. This could give rise to very complex feelings, made up of differing values at each level, and perhaps a reason why we may shiver or cry in fear or in pleasure.

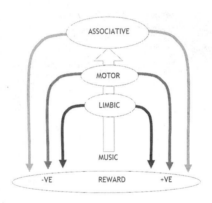

Three levels of reward

Although I do not fully comprehend the neurology of the malfunctioning reward circuits in Parkinson's nor can I relate it to my father's sad deterioration, I am finally able to think of the condition objectively, as the concept of three levels of reward loosely supports the model of my Performance Triangle.

How else can one understand a balance of physical, mental, and emotional functions if they are not all subject to similar rules of neural reward? Recent research into the subject of reward has three separated neural representations; wanting, liking and prediction of the same reward. [20]

This again makes me sure that three levels of brain activity are intimately involved in our pleasure of music. But how can we use this concept to explain this pleasure of music?

We need to understand more about emotions and music and their connections and also identify the attributes of music that generate wanting, liking and predicting and how they may be associated with the limbic, motor, and associative rewards circuits.

CHAPTER 6

Sweet and sour music

MORE THAN 2,000 years ago Aristotle wrote: "Why is sound the only sensation that excites the feelings? Even melody without words has feeling."[21]

When the MRI of my MS brain lesions prompted me to try to find out more about my brain, I wanted to know what exactly goes on when I create a stream of notes and why it gives me pleasure and how it is that I can make members of the audience cry.

I expected a boring, scientific exercise but, instead, it has become fascinating and exciting because I found that there are in science a few individuals who actively reach out to the general public in order to popularise their work.

In the field of music and science, I have seen the work of Daniel Levitan from McGill University (Montreal, Quebec, Canada), Edward Large from Atlantic, Anirudda Patel of MIT's (the Massachusetts Institute of Technology's)

NSI, Ekhart Altenmüller from Hanover, Stefan Koelsch from Berlin, Tim Griffiths from Newcastle, and Bobby McFerrin, who deserves a special mention for his amazing and entertaining demonstration of empathy with music but I am particularly indebted to Larry Sherman of Oregon Heath and Science University for his generous contribution.

The published abstracts and reports from the "neuromusic" scientific community are targeted at discovering the effects of music in specific areas of the brain. Using these neurological discoveries I have tried to understand and organise the musical functions of my own brain, to explain the very nature of music itself, that is, to break the code that gives us so much pleasure.

I have come a long way from my music theory and performance classes at the Gnessin Institute and the Moscow Conservatoire and realising the fact that pitch height prevails over so called, pitch chroma, altered my lifelong belief that emotions in music are linked to unique harmonics within the tonalities. I was left wondering precisely how music affects emotions if there are at least three neural pathways for reward and pleasure.

As I mentioned before, the question for classical pianists is: How does one create maximum pleasure knowing that music is partly instinctive, partly structured, and partly associated with emotional memory?

What appears to be fairly uncontroversial is the basic idea that music can trigger emotions, including happiness and sadness, and that it may even generate fear.[22]

This recognition of "emotions" being triggered by music can be explained by the concept of a combination of "arousal and valence"—the classic definition of emotion in psychology.[23]

Arousal is a physical and mental state of being awake or reactive to stimuli, involving the reticular activating system in the brain stem, the autonomic nervous system and the endocrine system, leading to increased heart rate and blood pressure, sensory alertness, and physical readiness to respond.

The human arousal state is demonstrated by brain wave activity and the range of brain waves Alpha, Beta, Gamma, Delta etc are defined by their frequency, simply put, the more aroused we are, the higher the frequency of our brain waves.

Valence is the subjective worth of an occurrence or simply a measure of our attraction or aversion toward a specific object or event that may be indicated on the brain waves as event potentials.

This presents us with a emotional model of high or low arousal with positive and negative valence.

The leading work defining emotions and music is the "Geneva Emotional Music Scale",[24] but I have arrived at the conclusion that this lexicon of emotional terms is limited by subjective judgements and a lack of empirical values.

The use of the scale as a scientific tool is restricted by this, and, indeed, the original forty-five steps in the emotional "scale" have progressively been reduced to twenty-seven and then nine steps that are now claimed as being a viable set.[25]

In fact we have not really advanced much since 1713 when Johann Mattheson wrote the following:

> "The composer has the grand opportunity to give free rein to his [*sic*] invention. With many surprises and with as much grace he there can, most naturally and diversely, portray love, jealousy, hatred, gentleness, impatience, lust, indifference, fear, vengeance, fortitude, timidity, magnanimity, horror, dignity, baseness, splendour, indigence, pride, humility, joy, laughter, weeping, mirth, pain, happiness, despair, storm, tranquillity, even heaven and earth, sea and hell, together with all the actions in which men participate. . . . Each and every Affectus can be expressed beautifully and naturally".[26]

These words of Mattheson described the main principles of the baroque "Doctrine of Affections" but made no attempt to specifically associate any "Affectus" with specific musical attributes.

Many scientists, philosophers, and musicians like Aristotle, Plato, Guido D'Arezzo, and Adam de Fulda have attempted to explain links between affections and music, but the results of their work are contradictory and incomplete, providing no definitive rules or valid explanation.

However, they all had one finding in common: They all believed that there is a function that associates music with emotions.

Returning to the Geneva Emotional Music Scale, I was interested to see that research has indicated that this scale and assessment model is not the most effective method.[27]

As psychology accepts that there are two elements in emotions—arousal and valence—we require empirical scales for both in order to permit objective measurement for the emotions in music. The current technique of asking a subject to select happy pieces of music for research and then playing them and then asking, "Does it make you feel happy?" is neither objective nor scientific.

The first person to define "valence" was Kurt Lewin (1890-1947), the German-Austrian psychologist. Lewin's equation of $B=f(P, E)$[28] states that behaviour (B; emotional response) is a function (f) of the person (P) in their environment (E), and the function varies in response to field forces that include positive valence that attracts people and negative valence that repels people.

Our emotions are the feelings caused by these forces, and their range has been described by the psychologist Robert Plutchik as eight basic emotions that developed evolutionally and other more complex emotions that should be seen as combinations of the basic eight.

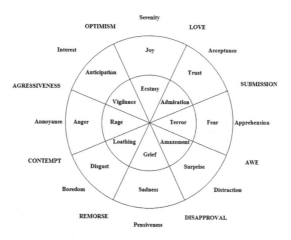

Plutchik's wheel of emotions

The model of Plutchik is not universally accepted, and there are almost as many versions of what are said to be the triggered emotions, as there are psychologists. The discussion about which emotions are basic and which are opposites can also serve to confuse any clear and rational thought on the subject of music and emotions.

It seems that our facial expressions may only represent four basic emotional states: anger/fear and sadness/happiness[29]. For me these might simply represent instinctive motor arousal and positive or negative valences, all other "emotions" being derived from interpretations of various combinations of the arousal and valence by cognitive or subconscious associations with our experiences in memory. This according to Rachel Jack, the author of the facial expression research, is similar to Russell's circumplex model and I think, fits the second level of Plutchik's wheel of emotions.

To simplify things, I take from Plutchik the concept of three levels of "emotion", and this I combine with Lewin's equation that states we respond to external forces in our environment.

Our emotional experiences as an audience seem to be caused by the combination of three levels of "field forces" of music in our limbic, motor, and associative functions, which in turn may involve three strands of reward: wanting, liking and prediction or learning [30]

The music itself was created as a result of "forces" and emotions that were experienced by the composer.

The objective of the artist it seems, is to recreate the field forces to both arouse and stimulate the valence of the audience's sensory functions.

CHAPTER 7

Another broken brain

I RECENTLY PLAYED A private concert that seemed to be well received by the members of the audience and I was pleased when I reviewed the recordings, which is a difficult thing for any pianist to say.

However, one important guest at that concert disturbed the concentration and silence of the audience, as he, completely disengaged from the performance, fidgeted and unwrapped sweets to pass the time. Subsequently I was told that he "has a problem" with music, probably having a condition called "amusia".[31]

Persons afflicted with "amusia" are very significant, as they are living proof that in the majority of people, the brain recognises something in the sounds we call music that causes us to engage and share pleasure.

To find out what those with amusia are missing in their brain processes it is necessary to identify what functions in the normal "musical brain" recognise the attributes of sound—as music.

When I play, my physical actions convert the musical score into sounds that the audience hear as music, and I expect this music to be interpreted into emotional meaning and enjoyment.

How is this achieved? What is it in the sounds that make it music? What is coded into music that gives pleasure?

When I read research into the use of cochlea implants, I found the basic facts regarding the "hearing" of the attributes of music.

For children with implants, music can be interesting and enjoyable and preferred to silence,[32] children were able to draw a distinction between "happy music" and "sad music".[33] While their perception of rhythm was quite good, they had more difficulty perceiving timbre, melody, and pitch[34] but improved in this regard with musical training.[35]

This work on cochlea implants defined for me the different attributes of musical sound:

- timbre
- rhythm
- pitch
- melody
- valence (happy or sad).

Understanding how the functions of the brain deal with these different attributes helped me to unravel the mystery of what music does in the brain. In particular it seems amusia may be a deficiency in pitch processing[36] associated with the brains white matter.

Keeping in mind that a "function" is something that "changes data" and that music's data is sound and its attributes, it was logical to trace these attributes though the functions associated with the limbic, motor, and associative reward systems. However, looking at the five attributes of music, it is evident that the starting point is timbre, the whole sound itself, as music is something we derive from a sequence of sounds.

The attributes of the timbre of sound are defined by:

- time
- harmonics
- volume (loudness).

These initial attributes are instinctively processed by the brain's functions to separate the stream of sound into:

- voices.

Each voice requiring an immediate survival evaluation.

The separated voices are then processed to decode motor signals from:

- rhythm
- pitch
- melody
- valence (positive and negative).

Finally, by association with our memory, the decoded elements are interpreted into conscious and subconscious

- meanings
- images
- feelings.

It seems that each of the functional stages—limbic, motor, and associative—involves the brain's reward system generating anticipation and pleasure and those with amusia fail to derive pleasure because they have abnormal or damaged music processing paths. I have a friend who describes herself as having partial amusia. She can obtain pleasure from some music with strong rhythms, but has no equivalent response to more melodic and emotional works.

This simple analysis of the attributes of music has allowed me to consider what parts of the brain may be broken in those people who miss the pleasure of music, but more importantly it provides a structure for any pianist to understand the separate elements of the processes of performance.

CHAPTER 8

Sounds in my head

WHEN I SIT at the keyboard to learn and practice or perform a piece of music, the last thing that comes into my head is the question, what my brain is doing? I simply trust that my brain will do the right thing. But can I help my musical brain to perform? Can I play in a way that supports the initial processing in the limbic system to sort out the sounds arriving as a stream of muddled vibrations?

The limbic brain considers our primal needs—safety, sex, and sustenance, and it would simply want to know where the sound is coming from and whether it is likely to represent a danger. So the initial functional challenge for the brain is to classify sounds to identify potential danger.

What does this mean for music? The immediate audio response at the instinctive level must occur quickly, in fact, in less than a second.[37] So the first strike at the keyboard and the timbre of the sound generated, triggers this first instinctive musical function and musicians need to understand that their first strike is significant to this processes of the brain.

Amazingly, we can recognise both an emotional meaning and the familiarity or non-familiarity of sounds in as short a time as 250-500 ms.[38] This explains how we recognise a member of our family or a friend from the first word of a phone call.

This rapid processing of emotional responses cannot be induced by rhythm, beat, pace, melody, or tonality, given the time needed to entrain a beat, enjoy a melody, or establish a tonality,.

Therefore, the immediate and instinctive "emotional" response can only be gained from pitch height and timbre, which provoke a level of arousal, an immediate valence, and an identification judgement in order to meet survival needs.[39]

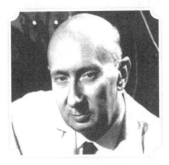

Georg von Békésy

Georg von Békésy, winner of the Nobel Prize in Physiology and Medicine in 1961, described the acoustic properties and output of the cochlea as encoded by frequency (tonotopic) providing for judgements of pitch height and timbre recognition.

The precise definition of "timbre" is the subject of much discussion, but the work of Professor J. F. Schouten who worked for Phillips industries for many years described the five attributes of timbre,[40] and his work was expanded by the American composer Robert Erickson in 1975 who described three classifications of timbre that range across:

- noise or sound without identifiable pitch tones
- sounds with a mixture of both with and without identifiable pitch, tones or harmony.
- harmonic sound with identifiable pitch and tones

These sounds are separated by silence or a background noise, have a start and stop time with rise and decay times and may also contain variations in frequency and volume like vibrato or tremolo. Research indicates that these different timbre characteristics are important for separation of sounds[41] into specific pathways. A function that identifies and separates sounds based on a ratio of harmony to noise has been established,[42] i.e. a precise location for the measurement and ordering of the three classifications.

So sound arriving in our ears has a timbre, a tonotopic quality and the audio processes of the brain have to identify specific attributes of this tonotopic content in order to separate sources of sound (noise, speech, music and so forth).

Imagine the differences between a flute in a quiet room, orchestral music in a noisy car, and a processed melody buried in techno beat.

I have a friend who produces techno music in a sophisticated studio and he has numerous contacts throughout the "club scene". We worked on harmonics, mixing, and rhythms, and I was astonished to realise that he could identify pitch patterns in techno music that I, as a trained musician, simply identified as a repetitive beat. Clearly the ability to extract pitch from the timbre of techno music can differ.

As the timbre is defined by the ratio of noise to harmonic tones, this allows judgements to be made about likely source and stress levels in sounds, providing a simple judgement of positive and negative, like or dislike, even fear or want i.e. an initial value of the valence of music.

So this initial basic information, from the first second of sound, it seems, must include both a valence (positive or negative) and an arousal state to support appropriate responses linked to our emotional feelings.[43]

The harmonic content, from total noise without pitch, to harmonic tones, it seems is the basis for valence and the brain response to this is positive or negative, representing: want—reject, like—dislike, acceptance—rejection, and so on.

Research indicates that the pitch of sounds relates to arousal in infants, who prefer high pitch for play songs and lower pitch for lullabies.[44] The pitch, extracted from the timbre is measured within our audio range, therefore can represent arousal; quicker for high tones and slower for low tones).

Trials to establish the optimum frequency to awaken sleeping occupants with audio fire alarms add a fascinating twist to the arousal argument. Specific frequencies may have maximum effects both for the conscious and subconscious arousal state.[45]

The possibility that conscious and subconscious arousal states may be linked by specific frequency not only indicates a concept that a specific pitch is the way into and out of an arousal state, but it opens the door to the concept that pitch height and arousal level are empirically linked. Such a link would allow pitch changes and pitch sequences to directly manipulate our brain through arousal mechanisms.

I propose that the first level of musical process reward uses the relationship of pitch height and harmonic content (timbre) for its decision. The dimension of pitch height arousal is represented by our audio range—for piano, the instrument range of 30-4,000 Hz.

We have a pitch norm of 500 Hz around middle C and a timbre norm of 50 per cent of noise to "harmonic" sound. The emotional vectors created by combining pitch arousal and timbre valence can be viewed as deviations from these norms.

It appears that asymmetric left and right amygdala rewards from the mass of matter inside each cerebral hemisphere, involved with the experiencing of emotions, may result from negative and positive arousals and valence signals.[46]

I believe that this initial survival-type "emotional" responses and rewards[47] provides an initial "emotional" response to music that can be represented graphically.

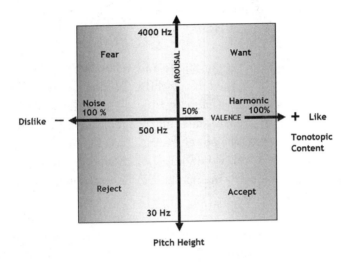

Tonotopic content versus pitch height

As most music is harmonic this has the effect that, most music is pleasing!

However, a key factor in this initial response to music is our existing emotional level defined as Pluchick's (PE) or arousal and valence, which may conflict with what we hear, explaining why we may or may not be in the mood for music. It is also the reason why Freddie Mercury entrained his audiences to his own emotional level before each gig.

As a performing pianist you must recognise that an initial mood is established by the arousal of pitch and valence contained in the first strike.

How we play this strike to create its timbre, should reflect an image of our meaning and demonstrate our mood for the work. Priming the audience to achieve a more common and sympathetic mood is worthwhile. This can be achieved by a few words, accurate programme notes of even a visual image.

I had discussed my ideas on this subject with a friend who is Professor of History of Piano Performance at the Moscow Conservatoire. He was interested, but he told me that if he tried to introduce the concept of verbal or visual images into the Conservatoire, he would be quickly removed from his post!

A few months ago he rang me to recount a discussion he had had with a senior professor of performance, a highly regarded concert pianist. This pianist had confided to my friend that he was having increasing difficulty with the first two chords of Chopin's "Scherzo No. 1 in b minor, Op. 20". These bars had become detached from the body of the work, and his stress was turning to paranoia, as he tried to strike these harmonically similar chords with any conviction.

Remembering what we had discussed, my friend gently suggested that he needed to imagine something as he hit the chords. Perhaps the crash as the aircraft struck the World Trade Center on 9/11 for the first, and, for the second, slightly less loud, a body falling to hit the ground. These horrific images provided a perfect rationale for the strike and timing of the chords written by Chopin to represent? "we know not what".

The result of this encounter was one happy and convinced pianist and a satisfied historian.

The first strike and all succeeding strikes generate continuous valence signals for each piece of music. Within this stream, the timbre of sounds is modified by time that defines the shape of sound packets: attack, decay, sustain, and release (ADSR in midi speak).

Timbre changes are not easy to achieve on the piano. Older pianos, that is, those made pre-1930, were built and set up with distinct low, middle, and high voices, but modern concert pianos have an even and consistent voice across the full keyboard range.

However, it is a fact that lower notes will have more harmonics than very high notes, and different attack and decay times, simply as a matter of physics, and thus they will have some difference in timbre.

As pianists we also create timbre when we strike chords, which contain many component pitches and harmonics. So, recognition of potential timbre differences and adjusting strike to highlight changes in timbre, is a skill that should be understood.

This is achieved by weight, speed of strike, and variations of timing based on some conscious intent that can vary the ADSR. The emotion associated with our conscious intent is the first thing that transmits to the audience.

CHAPTER 9

Voices in my brain

RESEARCH INDICATES THAT timbre characteristics are used to separate sounds into individual streams[48] with specific processing pathways[49] involving right neo-cortex and left temporal regions, [50] where these voices will be subjected to discrete linguistic and musical decoding.

However this identification and separation of voices is one of the most complex problems in the neurology of the auditory system, as it seems separation can be achieved by relatively simple criteria or by much more complex processing, using audio identification in the cortex.

As a musician that is passionate about voice representation in piano music I am interested in how this is best achieved.

The subject is called auditory scene analysis and the father of the subject is Albert Bregman whose book in 1990 "Auditory Scene Analysis: the perceptual Organization of Sound" effectively established the discipline.

One of his earliest experiments demonstrated that the brain can perceive or construct coherent streams of voices from a jumbled sequences of mixed sounds. Recent work continues to explain the mechanism of entrainment by which this is effected.[51]

While musicians may hear an individual voice in the orchestra, simply based on timbre, the same trick is not possible in piano music, due to the similarity of the timbre of individual notes, so for pianists the representation of voices is a challenge.

The secret of separate piano voices is clearly indicated in much research but not specifically addressed, as it is largely self evident.

The indications of research are: that sequences of similar sounds, can be demonstrated as separate. For me this indicates that voiced notes must be played as individual sequences, not coincident with other notes, to enable the neurology to function efficiently.

Notes struck in perfect synchronisation may be perceived as one combined timbre, so the introduction of small time differences between voices assists the brain in identifying and separating them.

But this reveals a cultural problem that has divided musicians for the last hundred years—that of musical voices and how they should be articulated.

The simplest voices of piano are the two hands, normally responsible for the rhythm and the melody.

Giving a master class at The University of Auckland in New Zealand in 2008, I was bemused when I asked a quite musical and competent post-graduate student, how many voices there were in a Rachmaninoff prelude. Like a young puppy with an earnest desire to please, the answer came back as a question: "Two? One?"

I was not really surprised, as voices are considered irrelevant and even an artistic mistake by many who do not understand the musical processes of the brain.

The concept of a leading hand simply does not exist for the majority of pianists, and voice management, to change lead hand or to introduce a third and fourth voice, to surprise and please the audience, which I consider fundamental part of performance, is certainly not valued as a competition technique.

Articulating different voices requires them to be separated by slight time differences, and this is the argument that has divided the piano world for more than one hundred years— to play hands apart or hands together?

As an "inmate" of the Moscow Conservatoire the biggest crime we could commit was "breaking hands". For the uninitiated, breaking hands is the technique that allows each hand to play independent, separate voices.

During my historic research into piano performance I found an article by Mark Arnest entitled "Why Couldn't They Play with Their Hands Together?" subtitled "Non-coordination between and within the Hands in 19th Century Piano Interpretation". Mark has analysed and timed elements of the recordings of most of the legendary old pianists and established beyond doubt, that the technique of putting time delays or grace notes between voices was common but progressively started to disappear a century ago.

I found the answer to his question why, in the words of Vasily Safonov, Professor of High Degree and Director of the Moscow Conservatoire from 1885 to 1905, in his book *New Formula*, published in Moscow in 1899. Safonov taught that we should consider the perfect equality of ten fingers and concentrate on velocity. He also is reported to have said, "It is unchristian (raschristannyi) to play with the right hand not knowing what the left hand is doing."[52]

This anti-Semitic statement, made for political reasons, seems to mark the beginning of the decline of breaking hands and also the decline in pleasure derived from piano performance.

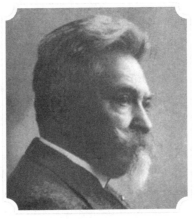

Vasily Safonov

Vasily Safonov, son of a Cossack general, was a career civil servant in the chancellor's department of the Russian Empire, but after six years' service he suddenly resigned his post in order to become a music student at the Saint Petersburg Conservatoire founded by Anton Rubinstein. He gained a gold medal in an incredible six months and in an equally short time, he became a piano professor and finally the Director of the Moscow Conservatoire.

In the State archives and on his marriage certificate, Safonov was still recorded as an employee of the chancellery while working as an assistant professor at the St Petersburg Conservatoire.

In these pre-revolutionary times in Imperial Russia, when students were involved in the plots of "Freemasons, Germans and Jews", it is almost certain that Safonov was planted in the Moscow Conservatoire in order to discover and eliminate disruptive influences and enforce Russification.

He spread his new piano doctrine through control of the Anton Rubinstein international piano competitions. These competitions created the pressure of zero errors and unemotional, risk less performances. These techniques coincided with the demands of the embryonic sound recording industry for perfection and speed, to fit maximum music in each brief recording. His most successful acolyte was Joseph Levin whose elegant but emotionless delivery you can find on YouTube. The skills of perfection and speed were rewarded above individual interpretation, until we finally arrive at modern performance where separation of hands and musical pleasure has been largely replaced by "shock and awe".

Safonov's new formula was driven by a number of things, first, by his own inability to play concert piano, in spite of his gold medal. He quickly changed to conducting, at which, Tchaikovsky reports, Safonov was initially completely incompetent.

The second reason for his formula was his quest to grow the number of students and establish standard teaching methods at the Conservatoire. Teaching broken hands, is very difficult and many pianists can never master the technique. By eliminating this style a larger number of standardized student could be produced.

Third he used the formula to challenge and control the "old guard of foreign professors" and their loyalty to the (largely German and Jewish) Romantic broken handed style.

Into this conflict Safonov appointed a young Ferrucio Busoni, the Italian virtuoso who he believed would support his case. Busoni reports that Safonov was supportive but that the existing professors did not accept him.

That is exactly how it would appear, except that Busoni was not aware that he was being used to cause trouble and that behind his back Safonov called him "Bezruccio Pustoni", in Italianised Russian, meaning "no hands and empty brain".

How wrong he was, Busoni was a strong advocate of voices. Simply read his preface, written the year he left Moscow, to the *Two and Three Part Inventions* by J. S. Bach where he criticises "the average system of musical instruction"[53] for not using the works of Bach as they were intended, that is, to fully explain and teach the writing and performance of two and three voices.

I warm to Busoni for two other reasons: first, his wonderful arrangements and second, as a dog lover.

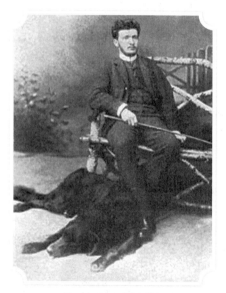

Busoni and Lesko

In 1888, in Leipzig, Busoni got Lesko a Newfoundland dog who was much-loved, and they became inseparable and moved together to Helsinki in Finland and then to Moscow. After his short and unhappy stay in Moscow during 1890 and 1891 Busoni moved to America and was forced to leave his beloved Lesko behind, with none other than, my ignored Paul Pabst and his wife Alexandra Petrovna.

When Busoni returned to Moscow four years later, he wrote to his wife Gerda:

> "A sad news, Lesko died quietly four weeks ago.
> He was called and did not answer, they thought
> he was asleep, shook him but he did not move,
> he was dead. Pabst really loved him and treated
> him well and he cried when he died.[54]

This touched me so much, as it describes exactly the death of my own beloved black Alsatian, Gipsy.

In a final echo from canine musical history, Rachmaninoff called his beloved, identical-looking Newfoundland dog Levko. The similarity of name and pictures leave me speculating on the musical and genetic connections.

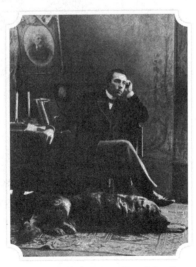

Sergei Rachmaninoff and Levko

But returning to the twenty-first century, a final comment of voice separation is made by the biggest selling pianist on the planet, Richard Cleyderman, so criticised and despised by the musical literati.

When he plays his massive hit "Ballade for Adeline" as a piano solo, he breaks hands in spectacular fashion,[55] in a manner that is truly "*raschristannyi*".

You may argue with me the benefits of voice separation and management, but in doing so you take on J. S. Bach and his acolytes Albert Schweitzer and Ferruccio Busoni and the neurology of the brain.

I am confident I am on the right side of the argument and that voice separation is a fundamental part of all styles of music.

To argue that voices do not need to be separated is both illogical and ignorant. Why do composers write separate voices, if they don't intend them to be played?

CHAPTER 10

"First there was rhythm"

AFTER THE FIRST few hundred milliseconds, our limbic system provides for separation of sound by timbre and time into voices with discrete paths in the brain for further processing. So what happens next, in the middle section of the brain with its motor reward circuit?

The sound stream by definition, is a series of sounds with pitch attributes divided by time intervals defining the pace and rhythmic attributes. How does the brain make sense of the basic pitch and pace of music or language?

Hans von Bülow, the legendary pianist and the founder of the Berlin Philharmonic orchestra, is credited with the musical quotation: "First there was rhythm."

As fashions in music come and go, rhythm is the common mark that they leave on history: Passacaglia, Waltz, Foxtrot, March, Swing, Charleston, Jive, Rock 'n' Roll, Cha-cha, Twist and so on.

This human love for rhythm seems to be a natural expression of a brain function: our ability and need to listen, learn, imitate, and anticipate. This may be so, but considering the audio system as a sensory device, it is evident that the brain needs to make sense of all of the data carried by sound. What we call rhythm is simply a very low frequency event when compared to the sounds of the audio range.

Regular audio patterns in the cortex trigger responses in the brains motor system and this leads to entrainment[56] [57] of the rhythm or pace of the music, as we instinctively join in with the beat.

This action of entrainment can vary the heart rate and at the same time our physical levels of arousal.[58]

While is difficult to immediately pick up a very fast beat, it is easier to be entrained to a beat close to our current arousal and then to be moved to higher arousals by increasing pace.

It is not so simple to demonstrate exactly how and why we can entrain to different beat patterns, such as:

- the beats per minute indicated on a score
- the rhythmic pattern (time signature) the 3/4 Waltz, the 2/4 Polka, and the 4/4 March
- the slower "alla breve" half beat or beat on the bar.

Our differing responses may represent differing arousal states in the audience.

We do, however, seem to be able to recognise and combine rhythms when the period can be demonstrated as harmonic. In fact, we divide musical time by two, four, eight, and sixteen, which are easily combined, but the principle of musical time is that, both even and odd numbers of beats will combine by the end of the bar, allowing weird time signatures like 11/4 used by Rimsky-Korsakov in the opera "Sadko".

I witnessed a massive experiment in entrainment at the Verona Arena, when an audience of approximately 20,000 people suffered a very poor "Domingo Gala Concert", constructed for "academic reasons" to celebrate the 200th anniversary of the birthdays of Verdi and Wagner who, incidentally, hated each other and each other's music.

To arrive in Verona, the heart of Italian music, to find that the programme was to be two-thirds' Wagner, was an insult I will never forget.

Maestro Domingo I think, sensed the audience's disappointment and frustration, and, as an encore started, he snatched the baton from Daniel Harding and conducted the Anvil Chorus from "Il Trovatore" himself. The effect on the audience was simply electric; from the second beat, the entrainment started until the whole auditorium was clapping their chosen beat by four or "alla breve". I was fascinated by two things: the differing beats entrained in the audience but mainly the effect of the different conductor.

It seemed to me, that after two hours of notes, the music had finally started with this impromptu encore by Maestro

Placido, who incidentally was recovering at the time, from recent heart surgery. Sadly it was the only memory I took away, from what should have been an iconic event.

It is possible to guarantee instinctive entrainment by an audience using particular works: The Russian song "Kalinka", Rossini's "William Tell Overture", or "The Entertainer" by Scott Joplin nearly always achieve results.

The secondary effect of rhythmic entrainment is that we identify patterns associated with memory, for example, dance rhythms that may be remembered as images of dancers or ourselves dancing.

It is my personal experience that entrainment is easiest when it reflects natural human timing, in techno music, the best hits are generated by mixing clips of live recordings. Something seems to be missing from recordings using only computer-generated rhythm and beat.

However, the subject of brainwave entrainment is considerably more complex than simply clapping to a rhythm.

There is a growing industry based on therapeutic claims about manipulation of Theta and Alpha waves using "shaman drumming" techniques or combining musical tones to generate low-frequency binaural or monaural beats that seemingly entrain the various brainwaves.

Looking for specific research into the simple phenomenon of musical beat and arousal was quite difficult; perhaps we all just assume that it happens.

However, the search was worthwhile, revealing that the tempo of music does induce arousal effects, and slow music or pauses, induce a relaxing effect, with an associated reduction in blood flow in the mid-brain in direct correlation to beat.[59]

To add to this finding, it appears that arousal itself is linked to brainwave propagation; hence a mechanism exists for beat-based arousal to change brainwave patterns.[60]

A practical demonstration of this effect has been described in music therapy where a 69 bpm rhythm was effective in reducing adverse symptoms in children with autism.[61]

The work of Joel Snyder and Edward Large has probed this concept by indicating connections between gamma wave activity and response to rhythmic tones.[62]

But rhythm alone, while it can arouse and provide entrainment reward, does not have an emotional content, it seems that another attribute is required in order to establish valence and this second attribute is, I believe, pitch.

Research demonstrates that in the voice stream, successive pitches are compared to provide up and down reference, higher or lower notes, which connect to positive and negative emotional judgement,[63] indicating a valence function associated with pitch.

As a musician I instinctively understand the difference between a funeral march and a happy dance: One is low and slow; the other is high and quick and it seems that arousal and valence combinations impact the functioning of memory, demonstrated by research into television viewers cognitive and memory performance.[64] But that is part of the processes of third functional level.

But first is it possible that we may be able to calibrate the arousal and valence response at the second functional level?

If we visualise a pitch range of 30-4,000 Hz, the full eighty-eight keyboard, and the physical arousal of beat to be represented by a range of 40 to 150 bpm, the range of both heartbeat and metronome, then we can plot their emotional relationship.

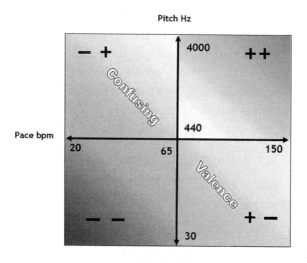

Pace versus pitch

Entrained rhythm is given as the arousal axis and pitch height is given as the axis indicating positive and negative valence, allowing pace and pitch valence vectors to be plotted.

This "double" arousal process reinforces instinctive valence of the limbic reactions, adding the second "emotional" level as indicated by Robert Plutchik in accordance with Lewin's theory.[65]

The neural basis of this function is the subject of recent research published just as I was in the final stages of editing this book. The thalamocortical mechanisms and brain location for the task of integrating rhythm and pitch has been identified.[66]

These external "field effects" of pace and pitch are affecting, they change our existing state, modifying how we feel. So the simple and self-evident lesson for pianists is: Playing quicker and higher makes a positive vectors, and playing slower and lower makes negative vectors and ambiguity is created when we play a combination of lower and faster or higher and slower, opening the door to a range of more complex emotions.

We also have the matter of tonal shifts rather than simple pitch variations to consider, but that comes later.

If the emotion in music is expressed at the motor level in terms of arousal and valence, driven by changes of pitch and pace, it is evident that as the composer has absolutely fixed the pitch by defining the notes to be played, the only parameter left for the pianist to manipulate is pace and expressive timing. Even though the composer has indicated the time framework, the relative length of notes and so on, the pianist is allowed overall judgement of pace and expression.

This allowance for human expression is the essence of performance; it completely governs the relationship with the audience, expression is our body language, the timing and touché that convey our human feelings. But remember we started in this chapter, with separated voice streams, each subjected to similar brain processes. It is possible that different voices may contain different pace and pitch data.

Muddled voices without clear articulation may confuse and fail to engage the brains of the audience. This applies as much to the production and conducting of orchestral music as to piano.

It therefore follows that clearly separated voices, fully articulated rhythms from a lead voice, play a key role in creating the maximum clarity for the brain processes.

Having argued for the basic emotional mechanism we are now left with the more complex questions for the brain: What made the sound? What does it mean? How does melody affect us?

The answers to these and other questions need to be based on more than the instant limbic reaction or automatic motor processes. Extra information is needed, such as pitch patterns of each voice of the sound stream to feed the cognitive processes of the third, associative level.[67]

But to complete our understanding of the motor functions and to even start considering associative functions we need more knowledge of music itself.

As musicians, we have an universe of knowledge: rules of solfeggio, followed by music theory, harmony, polyphony, art of fugue, musical forms, orchestration and composition.

Yes, to achieve our qualification, we musicians suffer nine years of hard labour without any promise that it will help us to perform and without any real explanation as to what it all means.

What is the magic of a series of tones that we call music?

How does the brain select which tone or pitch to process, when multiple voices, melodies, scales, and tonal shifts arrive from our two ears?

How and when do we learn to enjoy music?

CHAPTER 11

The chroma illusion

R EADING THE WORK of Diana Deutsch, it is evident she believes that we begin to learn speech and music in the womb and that the skills involved have common features. But Deutsch's work also raised a number of interesting observations about musical hearing anomalies, paradoxes, or illusions [68] that indicate the complexity and ambiguity of the functional processing of music.

The octave illusion demonstrates that right- and left-handedness can affect how octave-separated tones are perceived when played continuously through headphones.

The scale illusion also involves sound input through earphones to the left ear and the right ear, but this time, alternating notes of rising and falling major scales are split between the left and right ears. The brain perceives a complete scale rising in one ear and falling in the other. This effect is not changed when the sound inputs are reversed.

Other anomalies include the tritone paradox, which is an auditory illusion that confuses the up-and-down sensation.

Finally the chromatic illusion where the patterns shown below are played.

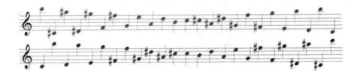

Chromatic illusion (played)

The illusion allows many subjects to hear two chromatic scales, one high and one low.

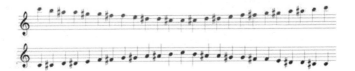

Chromatic illusion (heard)

In fact the brain is able to create an illusion of song from simple speech[69] and this strongly indicates that music and speech have common functions.

The summary of these illusions indicate that when our audio-processing system combines differing inputs from the two ears, we can perceive ambiguous results. Looked at another way, the separate pitches from each ear share a single common processor for octave and scale, and this leads to uncertainty.

Interesting though this may be, I am still trying to understand how a baby learns to speak with a high voice, while learning language from a father or mother with voices that may be octaves lower than the baby can produce.

Combine this basic problem with the anomalies and it is evident that there are many problems for baby to unravel: the timbre of the voice (its sweetness) that varies with pitch and physical stress, allowing differentiation of anger and happiness, regardless of pitch, as well as the ability to recognise similarity of sounds in different octaves, that is, identifying the chroma.

Seeking a definition of "chroma" I have read extensively, and the more I read, the more I became confused and frustrated. Musicians seem to have invested in the word "chroma" an almost metaphysical power, pretending that a particular key signature possesses a chroma with colour associations and emotional value.

The child's audio process for extraction of pitch or tone of voice from sound face a number of challenges. The first is the octave interval and the concept that all Cs sound the same. In processing terms this appears logical, as they are a simple harmonic progression identified by a natural harmonic function of division by two.[70] Presumably human physiology evolved around these physics of sound waves.

The neurological mechanisms relating to the octave are not clearly identified except that it is believed the process is located in the mid-brain, in or between the inferior colliculus (mass of nerves) and the medial geniculate nucleus of the thalamus,[71,72] where an octave function identifies audio similarity of pitches in the same class or chroma.

The ability to identify chroma is necessary for a baby to learn to speak or sing. This fundamental ability allows babies to imitate their fathers and learn to speak the same words at a different pitch. It is worth pointing out that, while humans have significantly different vocal ranges, their auditory range is effectively standardised.

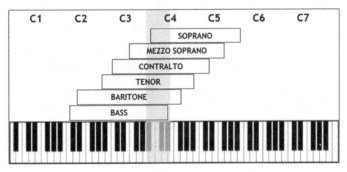

Human vocal range

But the vocal range of the singing voice is much wider that that for speech. A typical adult male will have a fundamental speech frequency from 85 to 180 Hz, and that of a typical adult female from 165 to 255 Hz.[73 74]

Exactly how and when does an infant understand that its high-pitched sounds mean the same as its mother's and father's lower sounds? Does this occur as part of developmental learning or is it instinctive?

I recently watched with fascination a three-year-old boy's first interaction with a man with a low-pitched voice. The game that followed, with the man making low noises that the three-year-old tried to copy, going as low as possible, all ended in laughter, and the boy finally found his own pitch to mimic the man's voice. This little episode suggests to me that babies actually have to learn to use the chroma capability, as a pre-speech skill. In the case of this young boy, while he was empathetic he had failed to learn even his first words of speech. Incidentally his mother has a extraordinary high pitched voice and excessively fast delivery.

Auditory physiology, convention, stylistic rules, nurture, and nature have provided us with the convention of C4 or A3 being at the centre of our musical universe. C4 or A3 is also the approximate centre of the tonal range of the human species, being within the scope of all voices, deep bass to shrill treble, making this octave of "middle" C the centre of our human vocal communication and tonal world.

The design of the piano keyboard reinforces this architecture; the pianist is effectively placed at middle C with his or her left hand and right hand either side and the expectation to go up to the right and down to the left. In musical notation this is presented by the bass clef and treble clef being divided by middle C, with the notation representing the tone ladder, going up and down.

From the illusions of Diana Deutsch I learned a fundamental lesson: "handedness" must play a significant role in music, as the musical processing paths include mixture of binaural, monaural, and lateral functions. Certain functions responding to left and right ears, and certain functions addressing the left or right hemisphere of the brain, particularly our handedness.

For a performing pianist this is a crucial lesson, it is more efficient to learn voices separately, generally hand by hand (with possible overlapping), before we combine them. Then we will undoubtedly find functional conflicts, but the decision to allocate priority to a leading voice or deliberately play hands together, should resolve any contradictions.

Taking this one step further, I remember a television programme[75] about a patient whose brain hemispheres were effectively separated, creating permanent conflict between the patient's hands, which appeared to physically fight each other, demonstrating the need for a function to manage priorities.

But a paper that opens up a fascinating concept was written by Bruce Morton[76] who proposes the concept of the "unilateral brain executive" being located in either the left hemisphere or the right hemisphere of the brain and that this is part of our genetic inheritance. He argues that left- or right-executive location causes bias of our brain functions towards the governing hemisphere, and this has some very basic effects on character and ability. In simple terms it makes us linguists or dot-joiners, but this theory is controversial.

However, logic must eventually vindicate the theory, as the evidence is all around us. We all recognise that list-oriented, methodical people with linguistic skills are different from more emotional, instinctive, intuitive personalities, and left- and right-handedness is unambiguous.

Confusion and controversy may occur because some people are ambidextrous, and many people show no real preference for linguistic or intuitive skills. Nearly every function involves both hemispheres, and people who have had one hemisphere removed can function nearly normally.

So if each side of the brain is fully capable, which side decides?

The theory does not interest me as much as observation of the practical demonstrations of handedness, and I am fascinated to look for evidence of left or right polarity in performers, including my students, but particularly in performing composers.

The ultimate musician needs to be ambidextrous and have both sides of the brain developed in order to combine musical and linguistic abilities that reside in opposite hemispheres.

Ignoring acoustic illusions and the possibility of left- or right-brain dominance, we know that we have a harmonic processing function at the core of our musical ability to make sense of pitch height and pitch chroma.

Not only do we learn the pitch class trick, but we also learn to mimic the harmonics of timbre in speech, independent of absolute pitch. We process pitch height and then pitch class (chroma) and then pitch intervals of scale and melody separately and this provides the ability to hear and reproduce a similar "tone of voice" at different pitch heights.

The tone of voice is something we begin to learn in the womb, demonstrated by our preference for mother voice as we learn the music of language and the language of music, but what precisely is a tone of voice in the restricted pitch range spanning less than two octaves 85 Hz to 255 Hz approximately F2 to C4?

CHAPTER 12

"It was not the words, but the tone"

THESE WORDS, WRITTEN by Tchaikovsky 135 years ago,[77] when his first piano concerto was rejected by Nikolai Rubinstein, the greatest pianist in Russia, made me realise that words are secondary to tone of voice when delivering meaning in speech and that is exactly the same for music, where the tonality also changes the meaning of melody.

The letter to Nadiezhda Von Meck in January 1878 actually led to the revelation that Tchaikovsky seems to have had help, to complete this controversial work, which has become the most famous and most recorded piano concerto in the world.

The insistence on the tone of voice to describe the reaction of Nikolai Rubinstein when Tchaikovsky first played his B_b concerto, indicated that Nikolai did not believe that his close friend Tchaikovsky had written the concerto and accused him of stealing it. He also provoked Tchaikovsky by suggesting that the piece was unplayable and trite.

Thinking about Tchaikovsky's words—"it was not the words, but the tone"—helped me by a comparison between music and speech, to fit together the pieces of the musical jigsaw of pitch, chroma, scale, tonality and emotions. The tone of speech is simply a natural reflection of, or deliberate projection of, feelings that we wish to generate in the listener and that, most importantly, must be understandable regardless of pitch class height, to allow high or low voices to express similar emotions.

In speech the variations indicating emotions are described as prosody, when we start a sentence, we choose a pitch and a pace that reflects an arousal level and valence that is, on its own, an emotional statement. As the sentences or phrases progress, the pitch rises and falls, indicating changes of arousal/valence, until the last pitch, which can be neutral, high, or low in order to convey the final emotional message.

The next sentence or phrase will also have a starting pitch or pace, one that is either linked to or distinct from the previous ending. The tricks of the orator use tone and pace to arouse the members of the audience. Remove the words, and language and music share common effects and objectives, allowing us to understand the "tone" regardless of the actual pitch height.[78]

What precisely is a tone of voice, and how is it connected to pitch class?

An angry baby makes a different sound to an angry man, as they speak in different pitch classes, but we still understand both the words and the meaning, when they use similar tones of voice. The range of the emotional tonal scale must be constrained within an octave and transportable thought the pitch classes.

If we consider the human larynx as a pipe, then it is evident that it has a natural resonant frequency and limited pitch range based on our ability to vary its effective length. However our auditory range is not similarly constrained and this allows us to process many pitch classes.

The natural mechanism for the production of pitch/tone is arousal or stress, resulting from emotional tension. Relaxation returns us to our natural resonant pitch and timbre, our neutral emotional tone. This means that our natural ability to create and reproduce tones is individually limited but to allow the species to communicate, the tonal values must in some way be emotionally interchangeable across the human voice range.

To be sure of the mechanisms of music we need to look at several things: pitch, the 12 tones of the octave, and the concept of scales. However, before doing this I will tell you the rest of the story of B-flat minor, Tchaikovsky's first piano concerto.

Perhaps the best place to start again is with Tchaikovsky's own words: "In 1874 I wrote a piano concerto and as I am not a pianist I needed help with the passages."

This tacit admission that he needed help has never been expanded on, and it has not, to my knowledge, been taken up by musicologists or historians. No one dares to criticise the icon of Russian music. However, I found the imprint of a second pair of hands through learning another musical work, a piano paraphrase of Tchaikovsky's opera "Eugene Onegin" that is dedicated to Nikolai Rubinstein.

My discovery of this fantastic piano work, written by the unknown Paul Pabst, prompted me to research the history of the period in great detail. I discovered that in October and November 1874 Tchaikovsky wrote letters complaining of how impossibly difficult he found writing the concerto. He finally decided to go to Kiev for the opening of his opera "Oprichnik", simply to get away from his difficulties composing the piano passages for his new concerto.

When he returned, less than two weeks later to Moscow, on 13 December of 1874 he told his brother Modest and others, that his concerto was finished and that he had just had "the best week" of his life.

This happiness was short-lived, however, shattered by the reaction of Nikolai who refused the work that Tchaikovsky had dedicated to him. This resulted in the world premiere performance of the concerto being played by a German, Hans von Bülow, in the Old Music Hall in Boston in the United States rather than in Russia, by a Russian pianist.

More than two years elapsed, and suddenly Nikolai publicly announced that he would play the concerto, which he did in Moscow, St Petersburg, and, finally, in August 1878 at the Great Exhibition in Paris, in the magnificent hall of the Trocadéro.

The confession to Nadezhda Von Meck, Piotr Illich's generous benefactor, coincided with the news[79] that Nikolai had finally decided to play the concerto.

Apart from my knowledge of all of Tchaikovsky's piano works, and evidence that the concerto is different, there are three facts that convince me that Pabst was involved. First, there is a statement by Kashkin in his obituary of Pabst that he was in the Kiev Opera in December 1874; second, there was the visit of Taneyev, Nikolai's favourite pupil, to the home of Pabst, in Riga in March 1878, in the same week as Nikolai's first performance of the concerto in Moscow; and, finally, there was the journey of Pabst to Moscow via Smolensk that coincided with Nikolai's triumphal return from Paris in early September 1878.

If you compare the various versions of the scores of this concerto, it is evident that the first published edition (1875) and presumably the manuscript as well (given Tcahikovsky's "I will not change a note") contains a huge error that prompted Nikolai's challenge of it being unplayable.

This error could only be explained if a non-virtuoso pianist had tried to transcribe to a score from what he saw a virtuoso playing at the keyboard.

The final act of this musical mystery is held in the Hermitage Restaurant on 22nd September 1878 to celebrate Nikolai's triumphant success with the concerto in Paris. As

Nikolai congratulated Tchaikovsky with the words, "It is not I that brought honour to Russia abroad. . . . [T]here is the man: He wrote the music; I only played it", Tchaikovsky reportedly "got to his feet, blushing like a girl, fled in embarrassment".[80] Within a week he had resigned his post at the Moscow Conservatoire, and Pabst was appointed as assistant professor of piano to replace Taneyev who took Tchaikovsky's harmony classes.

The harmony class is most appropriate place to end, as this is where we need to discuss the very nature and harmonic origins of music.

CHAPTER 13

In harmony with China

S EARCHING FOR THE origins of music, I found a confusion of flutes, scales, and theories.

The earliest musical artefacts are estimated to be over 40,000 years old—from Divje Babe near Cerkno in north-western Slovenia where a bone fragment from a Neanderthal cave, referred to as a Neanderthal flute, can supposedly play D, E, F, G (in a modeled version of the artifact). From rock shelters at Isturitz in the Dordogne where more than twenty flutes were discovered, dated to be from 20,000 to 35,000 years of age.

In spite of extensive theorising about their finger hole positions, no conclusive musical scales theory has been established for these remains. However, if we move to a tomb in Henan Province, eastern central China and forward to about 7,500 years ago, we have the world's oldest playable flute.

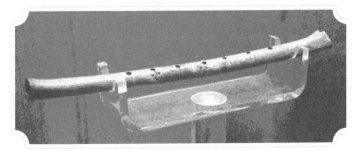

Ancient Chinese flute

It has seven holes at the front and one thumb hole at its back and can play four, five, six, or seven note scales, compatible with modern music.

Flutes from other excavations suggest that music in China progressively developed from using four to five and then six and seven note scales in a period of about 1,200 years.

More surprising is the fact that a complete set of bronze bells were found in the tomb of the Marquis Yi of Zeng from the 5th century BC. These bells cover five octaves with seven-note scales in the key of C major, including a twelve-note semi-tones full chromatic scale, in the middle of the range.[81]

This ancient multi-octave instrument demonstrates that very early musicians understood not only the octaves but the same twelve divisions of the octave that we recognise today. This argues there is something in our human neurology, that supports both the octave and its natural divisions.

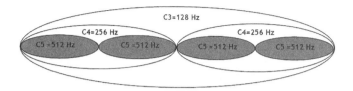

The harmony of the octave chroma

The natural evolution from the basic octave harmonics and the resulting pitch class relationships based on multiples of two, is a harmonic system based on multiples of three. The basis of these second level of harmonics is the relationship of 3/2 shown below with the additional harmonic of 3/1.

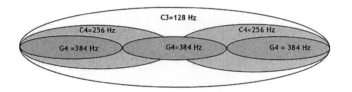

The harmony of the fifth

With the pitch interval increasing by half at each step or the wavelength reducing by one third, we establish a sort of "super scale" that is known as a progression of fifths.

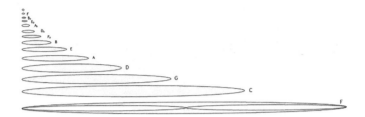

Super scale of the progression of fifths

In the table below very close to Mozart's tuning, the middle column contains the major progression of fifths intervals up and down from C4 tuned at a nominal 256 Hz. I have chosen 256 as it is easily divisible and multiples are easily identified.

				FIFTHS Hz 2:3				
				Gb 22.47	44.94	89.88	179.76	359.52
				Db 33.71	67.42	134.84	269.68	539.36
CIRCLE OF 5THS			25.28	Ab 50.57	101.14	202.28	404.56	809.12
		18.96	37.92	Eb 75.85	151.70	303.4	606.8	1213.6
	14.22	28.44	56.88	Bb 113.77	227.50	455.11	910.22	1820.44
	21.33	42.66	85.33	F 170.66	341.33	682.66	1365.33	2730.66
OCTAVES 1:2	C1 32	C2 64	C3 128	C4 256	C5 512	C6 1024	C7 2048	C8 4096
	48	96	192	G 384	768	1536	3072	6144
CIRCLE OF 5THS	72	144	288	D 576	1152	2304	4608	9216
	108	216	432	A 864	1728	3456	7512	15024
	162	324	648	E 1296	2592	5184	10368	20736
	243	486	932	B 1864	3728	7456	14912	29824
	364.5	731	1462	F# 2924	5848	11696	23392	46784

	Harmonically Arranged Scales											
Pythagoras		9/8		5/4	4/3		3/2		5/3		15/8	
Pythagoras		288		320	341		384		426		480	
C4	Db	D	Eb	E	F	F#	G	G#	A	Bb	B	C5
256 hz	269.68	288	303.4	324	341.33	364.5	384	404.56	432	455.11	486	512

Typical mathematics of the fifths

The fifth of C4 (256 Hz) is G4 (384 Hz), which is harmony with C3 (128 Hz). In fact G4 is the sum of C4 and C3. This super scale is repeated twelve times stretched over eight octaves.

The bottom line of the table contains the super scale transposed to the twelve semi-tones between C4 (256 Hz) and C5 (512 Hz) of our chromatic progression i.e. the twelve chroma represented throughout the octave classes.

The number of transpositions through the octaves indicates the closeness of the harmonic relationships. Starting at a nominal C we create fifths (arrows) and transpose into a single octave (shaded).

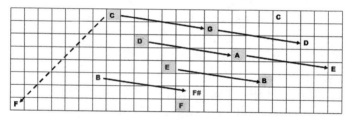

Transposition of fifths into an octave (1)

We arrive at F#, which doesn't fit our scale, consequently we seek F by measuring a fifth down from C and transposing up.

Similarly we populate the "sharps" starting at F#.

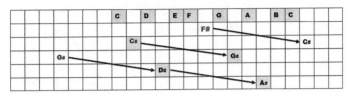

Transposition of fifths into an octave (2)

And the "flats" continuing downward fifths but transposing upwards.

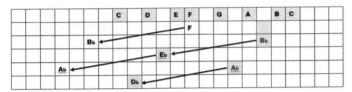

Transposition of fifths into an octave (3)

But it is evident that there is an ultimate discrepancy between the intervals calculated by fifths and the pitch class octave progression, demonstrated by the fact that F-sharp and G-flat have different values but on the modern piano are the same key.

These differences have provided musicologists with something to write about for hundreds of years, as they theorise about differences between Pythagoras and just tuning, equal tuning, the invention of cents, wolf intervals, and Pythagorean gaps, seemingly missing the point that Pythagoras simply developed a method of tuning, to achieve the frequencies that are acceptable to our neurology over a restricted number of octaves.

Endless papers on these minutiae miss the basic neurological facts that the twelve-tone music system is based on the fifths that fit our physiology and its natural appreciation of harmony understood in Ancient China where rich Chinese emperors could afford to commission sets of bells to fix tonal standards.

The more democratic Greek music is known to have been limited to simple stringed instruments or flutes. However, the Greeks as we know from their history, myths and archaeology, maintained a concept that music gives pleasure and healing.

I am sure you will be as surprised as I was, to discover that the old Chinese character for music is, 樂, a character that also means pleasure.

I had another surprise when I found that the character for a medicine, a drug, or a cure is the same as that for music and pleasure except that the character for grass/herb was added on top: 藥.

Is it possible that the long-held belief that combine medicine and music are based, in part, on the emotional values and therapeutic effects of rhythmic and melodic sounds?

CHAPTER 14

Music and medicine
of Ancient Greece

I ENJOYED *JOANNA LUMLEY's Greek Odyssey*[82] but was particularly inspired by her standing in the theatre of Epidaurus talking about medicine, music, and healing—and I knew that I had to visit this special place.

As with many things in life, a simple coincidence happened. I was invited to a musical birthday party in the village of Nea Epidavros, just five kilometres from the iconic archaeological site, and I booked to stay in a hotel at the little port of Palaia Epidavros, unaware of the surprises that awaited me.

As we drove south along the eastern Peloponnese coast, the landscape became increasingly green, and the valley joining the port at Palaia Epidavros to the theatre and temples at the Asclepios of Epidauros, was simply luscious with orange groves, vines, and olives. Some trees, of five-metre girth, must be many hundreds of years old.

The first surprise was that the little port has its own small theatre and a sunken city with archaeology stretching back into the Stone Age. The micro-climate creates cool breezes, and the horizon of islands that surround the bay is like a sunrise calendar, creating a feeling of security even in the midst of the current financial crisis.

The peace and strength of this place is reflected in the exceptional kindness of the residents. It seems so natural that this small harbour town, was a gateway to an ancient place of healing, centred in the temples at Epidauros, built by the followers of Apollo and his son Asclepios, on the site of earlier Mycenaean temples of 1800 BC.

Music it seems was indivisible with early medicine, and the word "Paean" refers to both the name of the physician to the Gods and his ritual musical spells. It is a word that became associated with both Apollo and Asclepios.

For me the most fascinating part of this history is that Epidauros seems to be the source of the doctor's oath and a place where music was used for healing. Due to its location in the heart of the Dorian region, it is possible that their scale was used to sing the therapeutic music.

The music of Ancient Greece, while it had links to medicine like Ancient China, was different; there is no evidence that the Greeks had a concept of twelve tones that the Chinese had by 500 BC, possibly because the concept of democracy required music that was playable by all, thereby restricting the musical standard to seven tones and pipes rather than octaves of expensive bells.

Hippocratic oath

I swear by Apollo Physician, by his son Asclepius and his daughters Hygena, by Panacea, and by all the gods and goddesses, making them witnesses, that I will carry out, according to my ability and judgment, this oath and this indenture: To regard my teacher in this art as equal to my parents; to make him partner in my livelihood, and when he is in need of money to share mine with him; to consider his offspring equal to my brothers; to teach them this art, if they require to learn it, without fee or indenture; and to impart precept, oral instruction, and all the other learning, to my sons, to the sons of my teacher, and to pupils who have signed the indenture and sworn obedience to the physicians[1] Law, but to none other.

I will use treatment to help the sick according to my ability and judgment, but I will never use it to injure or wrong them. I will not give poison to anyone though asked to do so, nor will I suggest such a plan. Similarly I will not give a pessary to a woman to cause abortion. But in purity and in holiness I will guard my life and my art.

I will not use the knife either on sufferers from stone, but I will give place to such as are craftsmen therein. Into whatsoever houses I enter, I will do so to help the sick, keeping myself free from all intentional wrong-doing and harm, especially from fornication with woman or man, bond or free. Whatsoever in the course of practice I see or hear (or even outside my practice in social intercourse) that ought never be published abroad, I will not divulge, but consider such things to be holy secrets. Now if I keep this oath and break it not, may I enjoy honour, in my life and art, among all men for all time; but if I transgress and forswear myself, may the opposite befall me.

In Greek culture the muses combined poetry, acting, and melody as indivisible elements of performance. According to Aristotle, muses were performed in different "harmoniai" that affect the listener

> "But melodies themselves do contain imitations of character. This is perfectly clear, for the harmoniai have quite distinct natures from one another, so that those who hear them are differently affected and do not respond in the same way to each. To some, such as the one called Mixolydian, they respond with more grief and anxiety, to others, such as the relaxed harmoniai, with more mellowness of mind, and to one another with a special degree of moderation and firmness, Dorian being apparently the only one of the harmoniai to have this effect, while Phrygian creates ecstatic excitement."[83]

The Greek seven-tone scales or "muses" survived being renamed as musical "modes" by the Romans and then moved to folk music and the medieval "Gregorian" style and, finally, to Western "classical" music and modern pop.

The different Greek modal scales are produced by simply starting on different notes and allowing them to suggest differing emotions or characters that are named after geographic regions.

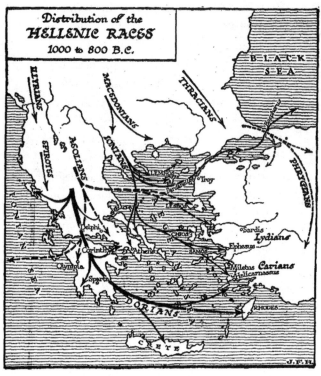

Greek musical modes and regions[84]

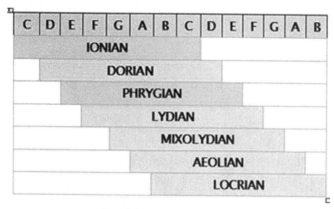

Greek harmonii or scales

This Greek system is not based on a series of evenly spaced tones, but harmonically compatible steps, for which Pythagoras gave us the first recorded mathematical description, presumably as a practical method of tuning instruments.

C	D	E	F	G	A	B
1	2	3	4	5	6	7
1	9/8	5/4	4/3	3/2	5/3	15/8

Pythagorean fractions

Invention, the development of instruments, and changes of cultural style had, by the twelfth century, allowed the seven-tone Greek scales to finally re-evolve to the twelve tones of the Ancient Chinese. The black keys of modern keyboards represent the tones that were added to the Greek system.

But because there is a basic flaw in the system based on fifths, F-sharp and G-flat have different pitch values, the progression of fifths does not fit precisely with the octave progression, so modifications were necessary.

With instruments having a small range of just two or three octaves this does not cause a huge problem. However, for keyboard instruments with five or more octaves, or the need for polyphony, and requirements to move between tonalities, the mismatch proved unsustainable, and adjustments to the Pythagorean intervals were made by the baroque musician Vincenzo Galilei who is credited with establishing the fractions of "just intonation". These were again modified in the time of Bach to equally tempered intervals by the master organ maker Andreas Werkmeister, each half-tone having common a ratio.

It was J. S. Bach who revealed the full glory of the twelve half-tones as equals, allowing us to move seamlessly around the tonalities, even if we are slightly compromising our neurological harmony.

But even in this universe we retained the limitation of the seven-tone scale!

CHAPTER 15

A world of scales

WHAT IS A "scale"? A "scale" is an ascending and descending series of tones that begin and end an octave apart. Tuning has nothing to do with the scale, as it is defined by intervals from the starting frequency. The series may vary in terms of pitch intervals or even the number of tones, and it can start at any pitch.

The evidence of the Zeng bells that shows an understanding of the twelve tones by the Chinese, that pre-dated by centuries the scales of the Ancient Greeks, it made me realise that the twelve semi-tones must fit human physiology, creating our natural appreciation of harmony. This means that the basis of music is universal, but we have simply adopted different scales from the twelve tones.

As early pipes were limited by the number of human fingers it seems that scales were practically limited to seven tones. It was accepted to have two fingers to hold the flute, one finger to stabilise or cover the hole underneath the flute, and to have seven fingers left free to play, and this became the basis of Greek and Western music. However, to follow the logical development of tones into the scales that are used around the world, requires precise terminology.

When I talk of "twelve tones" I am referring to what is now in modern music speak called twelve "half-tones". This is an unfortunate corruption, as the twelve divisions of the octave, defined by a scale of fifths, understood in Ancient China, that appear to be the neurological basis for music, should be defined as the twelve basic tonal building-blocks of harmony.

The next confusion is that we culturally consider seven tones to be a scale, and how we name the steps in the scale across the Western world is dependent on history and culture.

Until now I have used the scales C-B to describe the Greek system and its relation to modern music because this has the widest global acceptance. However, there are several names for our seven-step "tone ladder", which is the Dutch name for a scale.

Protestant	C	D	E	F	G	A	B
Catholic	Do	re	mi	fa	sol	la	si
Orthodox	до	ре	ми	фа	соль	ля	си
SCIENCE	1	2	3	4	5	6	7

Names of the basic Western scale

I have added, for simple understanding and use in science, a scale numbering system, of one to seven, similar to the

Nashville system invented in 1953 by Neal Matthews, Jr of The Jordanires.

This numbering serves to be the least confusing, as it fits with our definitions of the thirds, fourths, fifths and so forth, and it allows both easy transposition and comparison of scale systems and I use it as part of my teaching system to initiate very young, pre-literate students to the concept of scales and transpositions.

Within our western culture we have scales that are not simply seven tones. We have pentatonic and dodecaphonic scales, and I have discovered more than forty different scales from around the world that are based on the twelve tones we recognise as the full chromatic scale. The tables below show scales that use different numbers of steps: four, five, six, seven, or eight.

12	o	o	o	o	o	o	o	o	o	o	o	o	CHROMATIC
7	o		o		o	o		o		o		o	IONIAN
7	o		o		o	o		o		o		o	Western Major
7	o		o	o		o		o		o	o		DORIAN
7	o	o		o		o		o	o		o		PHRYGIAN
7	o		o		o		o	o		o		o	LYDIAN
7	o		o		o	o		o		o	o		MIXOLYDIAN
7	o		o	o		o		o	o		o		AEOLIAN
7	o		o	o		o		o	o		o		Natural Minor
7	o		o	o		o		o	o			o	Harmonic Minor
7	o		o	o		o		o		o		o	Rising Melodic Minor
7	o	o		o		o	o		o		o		LOCRIAN

Greek and Western scales

The first shows how Greek "harmonii" were forerunners of the Western major (Greek Ionian) and natural minor (Greek Aeolian) scales.

The second table indicates other seven-step scales that are known to be in existence around the world.

12	O	O	O	O	O	O	O	O	O	O	O	O	O	CHROMATIC
8	O	O		O	O	O		O	O		O			Flamenco
8	O	O		O	O	O	O		O		O			Spanish
7	O	O		O	O			O	O		O			Indian
7	O	O		O			O	O	O				O	Indian Todi
7	O	O		O		O		O	O				O	Neapolitsan Minor
7	O	O		O		O		O		O	O			Javanese
7	O	O		O		O		O		O			O	Neapolitan major
7	O	O			O		O	O		O			O	Indian Marva
7	O	O			O	O		O	O				O	Arabic Double Harmonic
7	O	O			O	O	O		O		O			Persian
7	O	O			O	O	O			O	O			Oriental
7	O		O	O			O	O	O				O	Hungarian Minor
7	O		O	O			O	O	O		O			Hungarian Gypsy
7	O		O		O	O		O	O				O	Ethiopian
7	O		O		O	O	O		O		O			Indian Hindu
7	O		O	O			O	O		O	O			Romanian
7	O			O	O		O	O		O	O			Hungarian Major

Other scales around the world

The third table shows the earlier scales based on fewer steps, presumably for simpler instruments. These come mainly from the ancient cultures in the Far East and Egypt.

6	o		o		o		o		o		o	Diatonic
5	o		o		o			o		o		Pentatonic Maj
5	o			o		o		o			o	Pentatonic Min
5	o			o		o	o				o	Chinese
5	o	o			o		o	o				Japanese
5	o	o		o			o	o				Balinese
5	o	o		o			o			o		Pelog Bali
5	o		o	o			o	o				Hirajoshi Japan
5	o		o			o		o			o	Egyptian
5	o	o				o	o				o	Iwato Japan

Older, simpler scales

The significant feature of these scales, is that they nearly all contain the eighth chromatic half-tone or the perfect fifth of Western music.

Regardless of naming conventions and ignoring the differences between the Ancient Greek system and our modern system, or major and minor modalities,

- How is it we perceive a scale and its sequence of notes?
- How do we know what comes next?

Our universal ability to answer these questions is in part demonstrated by Bobby McFerrin, who asks audiences to sing two tones in response to his jumping movements on stage and then induces a third tone from the audience simply by jumping to a new position.[85]

This experiment demonstrates the capability of our mirror processes to observe, learn, predict, and respond as an act of "entrainment". It works regardless of pitch height and across cultural boundaries. It is based on our ability to establish and follow rules using an inbuilt neural policeman that detects rule violations.

Functional MRI studies demonstrate the activities of a violation process[86]. The most basic rule violation being harmonic, the departure from a harmonically compatible sequence of tones[87].

The next violation being, deviation from a learned scale of tones and this is extended to violations of learned melodies. This opens a possibility for a rules hierarchy including learned rules of entrainment and basic natural harmonic rules.

A common jazz piano technique is the striking of two adjacent keys to create dissonance. In fact what is happening, is that the brain perceives and "beats" between tones, the two keys and the mid frequency. (Similar to the basic technique for tuning a piano). The jazz pianist is temporarily creating quarter tones, if a complete scale is played in this fashion, a virtual tonality is created.

This raises a number of questions regarding scales, pitch height, chroma, and harmony.

How does our brain understand which set of twelve half-tones we use to entrain a particular scale?

My understanding is simple: Our natural harmonic neurology, based on octaves and "fifths", provides the twelve tones that form a basic harmonic sequence recognised by our neurology from any starting tone, and from this we create and entrain different scales.

Indeed we have four scales in our normal Western music: the major and three minor. Each has a different emotional "feel" as a consequence of the arrangement of the steps, particularly at the end of the scale.

So the set of tones are defined by the starting pitch, and its resulting chromatic scale of twelve tones are defined by the steps that the brain accepts as harmonic, and, finally, the scale modality or contents is defined by a selection we have culturally evolved and learned like a melody.

Entrainment requires ability to detect violations of the scale rules in addition to our inbuilt concept of harmony and dissonance. This framework allows us to move between tonal scales like chess moves as described in Nabokov's novel the "Luzhin Defence". The trick of the composer is to turn the surprise of a violation immediately to compliance, by creating a new tonal context, this provides satisfaction for the composer and pleasure in the audience.

The magical part of the tonal system is that it works on any frequency or tone; we simply have to define the starting point.

Remember that Mozart's middle C was a different pitch to Beethoven's, and both are different to modern orchestral tuning. This calls to question the priestly qualification of perfect pitch: What pitch?

As the harmonic rules apply to every "pitch set or tonality", it is logical that the brain has a single harmonic processor and scale entrainment process rather than separate ones for every tonal set.[88]

In Western music the composer uses two ways to establish the starting tone: one, by using the first tone of the octave scale as the opening note, confirmed by the fifth (*a la* Mozart), and two, by demonstrating or resolving the fundamental chord (1+3+5) to indicate the harmonics of the tonal scale.

The illustration below represents the twelve tones, arranged in octaves, and the selection of tones of Western major is achieved simply by defining a starting point, there by establishing a new tonality across pitch classes.

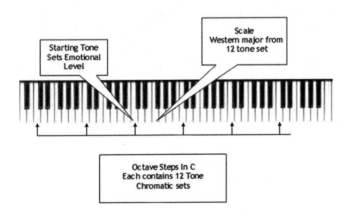

C pitch class, chroma, chromatic scale set

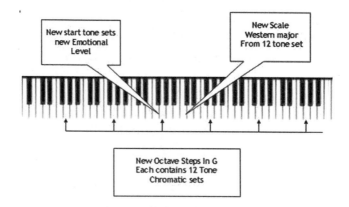

New start tone sets
new Emotional
Level

New Scale
Western major
From 12 tone set

New Octave Steps In G
Each contains 12 Tone
Chromatic sets

G pitch class, chroma, chromatic scale set

This new tonality establishes a new arousal level that itself has a full set of pitch classes or octaves.

This trick works simply because we reset the brain's harmonic processor at a new level.

Is it possible that we have ran out of defined terms and have run into confusion?

I read that we musicians can recognise both the chroma and the pitch height as separate things, processed in different parts of the auditory cortex.[89]

The conventional understanding of height and chroma is an elegant helix or corkscrew where notes of the same pitch class, that is, all Cs for instance, are aligned vertically and the notes of our Western scale progress as steps around the helix.

This does not make the scale itself on the helix a "chroma"; it is simply a scale demonstrating the chromatic feature of each step and this you might argue, effectively gives the whole scale a unique chroma based on its starting tone or pitch.

So I believe the enjoyment of music in all societies is based on human neurology and our natural ability to entrain scales.

Two recent concerts that I much enjoyed, provided me with examples of this universal nature of music.

First, a concert by the MED Orchestra, a group of Moroccan musicians, proved to be immensely pleasurable with their blend of Jewish, Andalusian, and Arab music—"Al-Alla-Andaluz", with its double harmonic minor scale.

Second, I heard music from Iraq in which very old traditions survive and blend with the modern maqam scales that include the use of quarter tones.

Without drowning in the minutiae of "cents" and "commas" and the mathematics of the inaccuracies and wolf intervals, it is evident that all scales, by virtue of their selection of steps from the basic twelve (half-)tones, have different intervals, that is, one, two, three, or four between steps.

These intervals themselves give rise to tension and emotional valence. I view these intervals as tone vectors that deviate from the basic twelve as the chromatic scale of twelve tones, while arousing, is even and displays no valence.

Scales with three, four, or six steps can be evenly spaced and fall precisely on the progression vector of twelve tones, hence for instance the neutral emotions of the diatonic scale and the nearly neutral feeling of pentatonic scales.

Scales with five or seven tone steps can only fall on the progression of twelve if they have unevenly spaced intervals creating vectors that cause tension.

So we have a musical "universe", divided into "galaxies" of twelve-tone octaves, each containing planets defined by scales.

But we created confusion, because the names of notes of our Western keyboard are ambiguous depending on their scale; for example, C sharp is the same black key as D flat. Creating even more confusion, F can be considered E sharp and C as B sharp or E as F flat and so on. I save you here from the discussion of the concept of double sharps and flats.

This duplicity is caused by the convention of naming the steps of all musical scales C-D-E-F-G-A-B, so some notes have to be designated either raised (sharpened) or lowered (flattened) in order to allow every scale to contain steps named only from C to B.

If the tonal systems are based on the natural pleasure and reward of our neurological harmonic capability, how do we explain acceptance of the dissonance of dodecaphony?

Perhaps we appreciate this at a more associative level which I perceive as a response to the disharmony of an industrialising society, world wars, and revolutions.

The great composers of the twentieth century selectively used the "disharmonic" elements of dodecaphony to illustrate the evil, inhumane, and chaotic nature of society, the most poignant example being Shostakovich's composition Sonata for Violin and Piano, Op. 134.

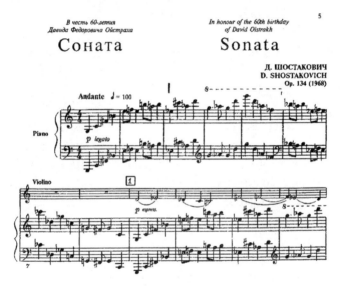

Shostakovich's composition Sonata for Violin and Piano, Op. 134

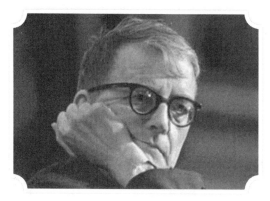

Dimitri Shostakovich

Thomas Mann, the humanist, describes the invention of dodecaphony in *Doctor Faustus*, his novel that he began in 1943 and published in 1947 as "music of the devil".

Just remember the early brain process—the evaluation of the ratio of noise and tonotopic content in order to establish an emotional judgement, and it appears we can accept and possibly even enjoy tonotopic dissonance.

CHAPTER 16

Prokofiev and Kandinski

THE ANNUAL MS gala concert in Brussels in Belgium is a fundraising effort. Last year a performance of Prokofiev's "Symphony No. 1 in D Major" was remarkable, and in the buzz of post-concert conversation, a comment was made that made me stop and think: "Prokofiev's music is like a Kandinski painting."

I had to agree that there was something that resonated between the pictures and the music.

Within days of the concert, Brussels was festooned with advertising for a fine arts museum exhibition of "Kandinski and Russia". Although there were only a few of Kandinski's own works in this exhibition, surrounded as they were by paintings and prints of his friends and contemporaries, I came away from the museum with new ideas about colour and the brain, prompted by a picture by a non-Russian painter and musician, Arnold Schoenberg.

I was struck by the dark misery of Schoenberg's pictures when they stood in comparison to the bright and optimistic colours of Kandinski's works, which seemed to change as his life progressed. In Kandinski's early works the colours are realistic but strong, and they gradually become more vivid. Then his palette changes to alternative colours chosen for their strong contrasts rather than their realistic effects. But through all of these changes the colours are vivid and arousing.

As his colours changed, his compositions also changed; from his early compositions of a slightly distorted reality, later becoming unstructured with confusing forms and finally turning into the precisely drafted strange forms with the bright colours of his famous last period.

These final pictures are like music—the colours having an arousal effect based mainly on their luminance, with compositions requiring mental deciphering.

The meanings of the combination of colours and form are derived from associations in the viewer's own memory. So the similarity between Prokofiev and Kandinsky lies in their brightness and the deliberate structures that provoke the emotional meanings. As they were cultural contemporaries, sharing war, revolution, life in Russia and, in particular, Paris, is it not surprising that they evoke similar memories.

By discussing painting and music it becomes impossible to avoid the subject of colour and music. This is perhaps unfortunate, as it is a subject that is full of controversy and very little science. There is a long history of theories of colours and music, and I am not sure there is any correct theory. But the discussion has value in the context of Synesthesia or the malfunctioning of the processing of sensory information.

Chromesthesia, the condition that causes audio tones to generate colours for a few special people, it is one of a number of conditions in which sensory information becomes confused. Scientific evidence appears to favour the possibility of cross modal interference.[90] There is no evidence of any general correlation between specific musical tones and specific colours between those with the condition.

Not discounting the fact that there may be some similarities between the attributes of music and light, as both are "energy" waves, sensed by our eyes and ears that become combined in some ways in the brain, I have tried to find some evidence linking light, colours, and music.

Sir Isaac Newton[91] aligned the spectrum of light to the seven tones of the musical scale, starting at D. Other eminent scientists, musicians, philosophers, and artists have claimed associations between musical tones and the light spectrum, from Fourier to Helmholtz and Scriabin to Rimsky-Korsakov, the Rosicrucians to the Theosophicals and even architect Edmund Lind.

One of the first physicians involved was Edwin Dwight Babbitt, who conducted quasi-scientific experiments in chromo therapy[92] and went on to misquote Newton[93] about musical scales and colours.

The most significant feature of this combined body of work is that there is simply no agreement between the experts. Newton and Lindt were the closest in their theories, as the difference between their musical light scales was simply a different starting point. Newton started at D and Lind at C, which incidentally was the only note that agreed with Scriabin.

Lind uses intermediate colours to correspond to the sharps and flats of the chromatic scale.

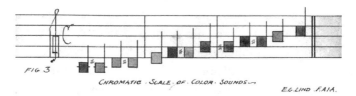

FIG 3

CHROMATIC · SCALE · OF · COLOR · SOUNDS →

E.G. LIND .F.A.I.A.

Chromatic scale of colour sounds by Lindt

The weakness of this science of music and light appears to be the suggestion that a specific note or scale has a specific or intrinsic meaning, that is, that C or D is in some way special. But the twelve-tone system is simply a harmonic progression, independent of its starting pitch height, so in theory, any sound may be any colour.

To get over this flaw, a new theory of the angstrom equivalent was created in order to directly equate the wavelength of light to the wavelength of musical tones of the octave C major, why C major I cannot imagine.

The theory goes that A=440 Hz and that is equated to an equivalent wavelength in angstroms/10 nanometres of

619.19, that is, that of orange/yellow light. However, there is again no correlation with other researchers, and there is flawed logic in the proposition based on the magical scale of C (whatever frequency that it is tuned to).

Sergei Rachmaninoff was dismissive of colour and music associations.[94] He wrote critically of the opinions of Scriabin and Rimsky-Korsakov on the connections between colour and music, commenting that the two composers could not agree on the colours.

I am quite confident in saying that there is no proven equivalence between any particular musical scale and the spectrum of white light. That is not to say that there is no logical argument for some equivalence between the harmonic twelve half-tones and the twelve colours made by progressions of our red, green, and blue perception. However, the choice of seven colours in the visible spectrum is flawed. The spectrum should logically be three or six or twelve colours, based on the combinations of our cone perceptions of red, green, and blue.

A six-colour scale could match a pure diatonic scale. A full chromatic scale could be matched to twelve colours.

But as any pitch can be the starting point of a progression, it means that any pitch may be any colour. But this doesn't mean that light is not arousing and that it does not contribute to valence.

The studies of chromesthesia at the University of California, Los Angeles (UCLA)[95] indicated the neural mechanism for arousal by light or the lack of light.

If one considers the structure of the eye, with its rods and cones, it appears that the rods that see in monochrome and that are effective in low light, are quite different to the three types of colour cones that are sensitive to long, medium, or short wavelengths that combine to create our full colour vision.

Could it be that vision's contribution to arousal is simply luminosity, and valence may be created by wavelength?

One of the most likely demonstrations of luminosity and arousal is seasonal affective disorder (SAD) where low luminosity becomes depressing, and the application of white light arouses and relieves the depression. Is it a possibility that valence is represented by blue short wavelengths being positive and that longer red wavelengths[96] represent negative valence while green middle wavelengths are simply more neutral and soothing?

One of the fundamental differences between sound and light is that we use sound to speak in real time, but we make very limited use of colour in direct human communication.

This statement does not exclude the fact that Kandinsky and other artists use colour to communicate and that there are notable uses of colour in day-to-day communication; for instance, we all understand traffic lights, where red instructs drivers to stop, and we constantly choose and use colours to suit our mood and sense of style in clothing and room decoration. We also blush pink and red and may go blue when cold.

I am still left wondering how the paintings of Kandinsky match the music of Prokoviev, as music moves and pictures are static.

But this discussion of colour and light does highlight the concept of the brain processing sensory information, by conversions to time signals, to be carried on our brain waves. In this context music may be used as a litmus test to calibrate other sensory information which it seems are implicated in many conditions like autism, dyslexia etc.

Assuming our sensory functions perform correctly, we derive instinctive emotional judgements from pitch and timbre, then pitch and pace, before the music arrives in the associative part of the brain, via our mirror/motor functions.

CHAPTER 17

Aristotle, Sting, and the mirror neurons

"WE FEEL THE motion which follows sound . . . These motions stimulate action, and this action is a sign of feeling."[97]

In spite of the clarity with which Aristotle, some 2,300 years ago, predicted the mirror processes of the brain, the mysteries of how "motion follows sound" and "motions stimulate actions" and the "action is a sign of feelings" are all still subjects of research today.

In 2006 when I wrote "Playing with the Mirror Neurons" there was still some controversy about their very existence. Even in 2011 I was heavily criticised by an eminent Russian neurologist who refused to even discuss the subject of mirror neurons. So it has been highly motivating for me to read many abstracts that claim evidence that proves that mirror neurons exist and that these neurons fire when we watch or perform an action, making them the basic mechanism for our automatic understanding of the actions and intentions of others,[98] that is, that they are a key part of our mirror/motor processes, our basic learning tools, at the core of our humanity. They form part of our instinctive and automatic response system, involving memory and emotions, their function being based on our need to "understand others". This means that when we watch a musical performance we use the "mirror" regions of the brain. However, this does not answer the key question: Does music itself trigger the mirror processes? It seems the answer to this question is a qualified yes: it is evident that music does evoke mirror response in musicians and non-musicians, various studies are quoted by Stefan Koelsch in his book "Brain and Music".[99]

In musicians the pre-motor responses are triggered though a playing response, and for non-musicians they are triggered through a linguistic or singing response. Interestingly it appears that there is also a basic tonal-matching mirror response. This is logical; how else could we learn to speak and sing unless we could copy sounds and harmonise?

This leaves us with two basic understandings: the first is that movement and sound can both trigger mirror responses, and the second is, that sound reception is linked to sound generation by tonal matching and mirroring. But any mirror responses require some memory for both successful repetition or interpretation of meaning. Music and memories with emotional meaning is a phenomena we are all aware of.

In 2003, precisely when I decided to become involved in music for MS, and as previously mentioned, I played an informal "lunch concert" for the European MS Platform (EMSP) in the Radisson Hotel in Malta.

As I sat and played "I Love You Olga", which is the aria from the opera "Eugene Onegin" by Tchaikovsky, a man in a wheelchair gradually approached the piano. As he stopped I saw the image of my father who had died from Parkinson's disease. In fact it was Daniel Carbolli who, for some reason, had tears in his eyes. As I carried on playing, I also started to cry.

This special moment demonstrated to me how music, memories, and emotions can link the artist and the audience, particularly when the members of the audience are physically close.

I experienced similar effects playing promenade events in Antwerp in Belgium and in Atlanta in Georgia in United States as people there also approached the piano emotionally engaged.

We have all at one time or another experienced the emotional effects of music, but precisely how these effects are generated is a mystery that is only just starting to be uncovered. Early and instinctive reactions to music[100] are only the beginning of a process.

Recently, on my visit to Epidauros, I met a music lover with spinal damage. Struggling on his crutches, he recalled one night in 1963 in the ancient theatre at Epidauros when the young village boys were used to scare away the noisy cicadas. He told me that he sat under the stars and the rising moon in perfect silence for a while, Then a single bird broke that silence briefly singing. To be immediately followed by the mesmerising voice of Maria Callas the Greek soprano. Fifty years later, the tears of joy from this memory, can still run down his cheeks.

This is without doubt the most powerful description I have heard of the power of music. How does this happen?

There is evidence that different parts of music provoke emotions: unexpected chords can provoke activity in the amygdala, indicating emotional response.[101]

However, when I read abstracts of articles about music and the brain, I was struck by two things: First, there appears to be no objective criteria for selection of the music for experimentation and second, the common use of orchestral music to investigate brain response is like trying to open a walnut with a road drill; there is an awful lot of noise and vibration and not enough precision. In Russian we have the saying: "Shooting sparrows with cannon."

The piano is an ideal research tool for neuro-music, due to its range, flexibility, and layout, which physically represents the tones and harmonics of the basic system of music.

Some of the more elegant advances at the McGill University in Montreal, and at the Atlantic University in Virginia in the United States were made using piano music and a Yamaha Disklavier, which allows precise objective calibration of musical input, using either live or pre-recorded tracks for comparison.

The apparent weakness of the piano for research is that performer body language and facial expressions are not easily observed by the audience. The seating position and the two-handed delivery creates a specific body language that may limit certain research aspects of the visual mirror transactions between the performer and audience.

For the audience, the visual elements vary significantly when listening to CDs or when watching a DVD or when experiencing a live performance.

Recent news items have reported a study from University College London (UCL) that indicated that sight has more influence when judging music than the notes.[102]

For the performer the studio has a different visual landscape to a live gig, and a need to read scores seriously restrict the visual landscape of the pianist.

Accurate and successful research of music and emotions using the piano requires the development of standards and an understanding of basic techniques, plus empirical methods for the selection of music. Performers need a technique to ensure that their performance movements are successfully interpreted.

The fascinating process of observing and copying is at the heart of our ability to learn. We obtain reward when we succeed, and even without guarantee of success, we try and try again.

From a superficial walk through research papers, I derive a simple theme that our physical body language engages and is engaged by, our mirror/motor responses,[103] and these are connected by mental processes to memory, which provides emotional meanings. In fact we empathise, and this not only justifies my "Triangle of Performance" but also brings us to the big questions: What is there to understand in music? How is it encoded? More problematically, how do our motor processes and memory contribute to the answers?

I was recently asked to review a research paper by Alexander Merkulov, professor of the history of piano performance at the Moscow Conservatoire who in a recent master class he was quizzed by a PhD student as to the rights and wrongs of movement at the piano when given criticisms for moving too much. He was also asked by the same student about the history regarding the movement styles of the great historic pianists.

Interestingly, after huge research into the letters, papers, and memoirs regarding the performances of characters such as Liszt, Chopin, Anton Rubinstein, Clara Wick, Scriabin and Rachmaninoff—all the way to Pletnev, one argument emerged: Movement is necessary in order to express music, but it must be genuine, that is, not movement that has been copied or falsely created.

Needless to say, Pletnev expressed the opposite view, that the greater the pianist the less the need for movement—a general remark that contained no references to music works.

To reach the conclusion that movement is essential, without science and without the other missing ingredient—the meaning of music, is a victory for common sense over current policy.

It is echoed in the words of Sting's famous hit that indicates that there is something more going on than simply watching.

"Every move you make
Every smile you fake
I'll be watching you"

How does the brain know what is fake?

Remember the recent study that indicates that sight is more important than sound in the judgement of music performance. For the performing pianist the lesson is clear, movement and your body language is part of performance, but it must be genuine. This raises questions: What is the body languages the pianist displays and how can we ensure that it is genuine?

CHAPTER 18

Footsteps in the corridor

W HEN I SPENT three months in the Russian National Neurological Institute and a Moscow clinic, I realised that I could recognise staff and visitors simply by their footsteps in the corridor, without seeing them.

Not only could I identify the person, but I could tell if he or she was anxious and in a hurry.

At the time this was not remarkable; lying in bed, in a restricted world, it was part of everyday life.

Much later, when my job involved buying and selling CDs, I listened to hundreds of recordings and used to play a game of "recognise the pianist" simply from the sound of his or her strike.

I also remember reading wartime resistance stories about how the Morse code signals were attributed to specific operators who imparted their own identifiable micro-variations in timing, thereby imprinting their unique characteristics into the signals.

This shows that both regular and irregular beat patterns are able to carry human identity information, meaning that the touché of a pianist is recognisable. This indication of our movement is the imprint of our own unique body language.

The scientific experiments of the "Perception of Human Motion"[104] have demonstrated our ability to identify the specific activity, the sex, and the mood of the subject simply from light dots that represent the human form in a dark room.

This recognition of the identity of persons from sound patterns and simple dots establishes a link between images and sounds by "cross modal transfer of emotion by music",[105] which suggests that music and images can share emotional effects.

The next part of the puzzle was quite stunning; I read that single neurons respond to more than one sense and that these neurons have direct connections to the pre-motor and motor areas of the brain. Not only did these neurons at the top of the limbic brain react to both auditory and visual stimulus, they reacted more strongly when stimulated by both.[106,107]. The concept of cells responding to both sight and sound, allowing our mirror system to respond to either visual and/or audio stimulation, may provide answers to questions about how the blind can empathise and how deaf people can enjoy music.

Reading further, I discovered the answer to my most worrying question: What do blind people visualise when they hear music?

It seems that we have a visualisation system that is multi-sensory, meaning that the blind can "see", and the deaf can "hear" by sensing neurological signals.[108]

Our body language can be interpreted by both seeing and hearing, a most logical function in human evolution.

These findings explain why I achieved such satisfaction and success with my performance genre "Live Video Music Shows", which combines the live audio of classical piano performance with custom-created video backgrounds. The development of the genre was instinctive and gradual, coming from my early ideas and reading about the mirror neurons and musical responses.[109]

I play a live "soundtrack", a technique successfully used by the MTV pop generation. Who can forget the images that were built to support the music of Michael Jackson's "Thriller"?

I took nearly three years evolving the concepts of music and image, starting by talking about images, simply to prime the audience with my own interpretations and then putting selected images in the concert programmes, and finally, creating slide shows and movies to be projected as I played. I have also watched with interest the first tentative steps by some major orchestras to try to utilise video background screens. So far, most attempts have been rather stilted and simplistic. Projection of video, allows real-time memory priming of the audience to be synchronised with the music.

To me it is very obvious that music primed by image is more enjoyable and more meaningful for the audience as it is more easily understood.

We all enjoy the soundtrack of movies and understand that music enhances the images, but my genre is the reverse: images enhance the music; if you have doubts just watch Walt Disney's original *Fantasia* (1940).

I have been constantly concerned, however, regarding the balance of music, video images, and my own body language. Am I still part of the visual show? If so how do I best integrate my natural body language, the back ground images and the music.

It seems that, even if I switch off the lights, my body language is visible through the ears of the audience. So for me the problem remains, how to integrate video, music and body language when all I have to control is my expression of the timing and loudness of the music.

CHAPTER 19

Playing with time and volume

THERE HAS BEEN little research into the volume of sound (except for its potential to damage hearing). However, many facts are self-evident: The volume of sound triggers the startle reflex and is responsible for some instinctive survival judgements about footsteps; louder steps are indicative of someone drawing closer whereas the sound of quieter steps are indicative of someone who is more distant, so increasing/decreasing volume can indicate motion to and from.

I have searched for evidence to support the idea that volume is directly linked to arousal, and the best I can find is that volume is a multiplier of other attributes. This is quite consistent with the normal understanding that changes in volume without a change in timbre can be ambiguous. A shout can be a shout of joy, of anguish, or of anger, rage can be quiet, a climax in music can be soft "*a la* Rachmaninoff".

This does not prevent us using our instinctive judgement in performance to provide meaning or dramatic contrast by using volume as part of emotional expression.

For pianists the composer's notations of forte, crescendo, and diminuendo give strong guidance, but it is necessary to understand the purpose of the instruction to play sensibly. Simply put, the pianist must consider what event or thought the volume change is trying to express.

For me, the most dramatic use of volume in any musical work is in Shostakovich's "Leningrad" symphony No. 7 in C Major, Op. 60; the slow building of volume is the main feature of the first movement.

So the rate of change of volume can be more important than the volume difference itself, but I find this difficult to consciously manage. I am often surprised by my own recordings and the way that volume changes have subconsciously found their way through my touché.

But volume of sound unrelated to time is almost useless; without time we would not perceive the slowly building drama. In fact, without time, music simply does not exist.

To identify the footsteps in the corridor, my brain calculated the timing of the paces.

Without time, nothing exists; the progress of time is the essential ingredient of everything we perceive, from the frequencies of light and sound, to the beating of our hearts, to the passing of night and day through the seasons and the years.

The progress of time is the engine of reality.

We accept and understand the essential regular rhythms of life; in fact we have audio mechanisms to exclude heartbeat from our auditory consciousness.

The irregular patterns in languages and music are all measured by time. We also make sense of our relationships through time, understanding the minute variations of moods expressed by others as they move, smile, laugh, and cry.

Although the need for time in the brain is self-evident, to enable us to both perform and understand the world about us, the precise time mechanisms of the brain are not well understood.

The discovery of a specific "time" neuron was a step forward, especially as it appears to be an element of the process of learning and performance.[110] The simplest of these learning and performing functions is the recognition of a musical rhythm or beat as the first task of entrainment. We need to measure and match intervals of time in order to identify regular patterns.

This brain time process seems to involve the basal ganglia, which is also concerned with the brain's mechanism[111] for providing reward following "anticipation".

But measuring regular beats is perhaps the simplest time task that the brain can do. Our survival and evolution needed more than recognition of simple beats; it depended on understanding the meaning of the more complex, irregular beats, so a process that allows us to identify sounds in irregular sequences is essential.[112]

But, for me, the crucial finding was that the same part of the brain was proven to be activated when one sees walking and when one hears footsteps.[113] This linking of visual and audio perception by time is fundamental, as empathy relies on our ability to link visual and audio perceptions of movement.

Research demonstrates that time and time processing involve a distributed network of several levels of the brain, from the basal ganglia to the cerebellum to the cortex performing tasks of storing and comparing time.[114]

Each of these levels requires some reward process for success. As we know, research into Parkinson's disease supports this by establishing that there are separate reward processes involving the brain stem, mid-brain, and cortex.[115]

So it appears that response to musical beat or time may be threefold; first, there is an instinctive physical pleasure response to regular beats in the brain stem, second, a mental arousal process causing changes in brainwave patterns, and, third, an associative timing process that allows us to identify the footsteps or strike so that we can identify which human generated the movement or musical sounds.[116]

Time is also encoded as part of other information, expression and images.

Musical expression is described in the work of Daniel Levitan's team at the McGill University who recorded and manipulated the timing between musical phrases.[117] Interestingly, timing variations proved more significant than volume changes, which alone do not appear to translate into emotional feelings.

Another interesting result of manipulating the timing of expression was that adding more time than the original, did not seem to add any extra emotion. It seems as if a genuine expressive performance has a built-in integrity that the audience understands.

As a performer, I sense that the ultimate empathy is synchronisation of performer and audience when we share the exact time for strikes.

I speculate that the act of human timing, that is, the choice of the precise millisecond to say or do something, is governed by the brain's rhythmic process, taking the concept of empathy from the emotional down to a mental level. This opens a possibility that empathy may include mutual synchronisation of brainwave rhythms.

The footsteps in the corridor give us some, but not all, of the information about the walker; I know that my own footsteps can tell others when I am tired, as my right foot drags a little, indicating whether I have taken my MS walking medication or not, but my footsteps do not typically tell the story of my urgency. Is my walk one of happiness at arriving, or is it a desperate rush to the ladies' room?

For the footsteps of the keyboard the same is true; pace and touch may tell of arousal and something about mood and may reveal the identity of the performer, but higher emotional reasons or images are more elusive, they require our cognitive functions, using memory and associative processes.

CHAPTER 20

"Memory, all alone in the limelight"

C HANGING A WORD in one of the most beautiful songs of the twentieth century describes my greatest fear as performer with multiple sclerosis. To be alone under the spot lights, with memory failure, unable to remember the notes.

The best classic story of a great pianist freezing on stage is probably that of Emile Gilels who, in a concert in Moscow, was to play Rachmaninoff's "Piano Concerto No. 2" when he totally froze on the opening passage and had to leave the stage, white as a sheet, to compose himself before trying again.

For pianists, memory is the essential tool of performance. Memory governs our basic ability to play. It allows our fingers and muscles to perform intricate patterns. It is the basic mechanism for recalling the music in order to ensure that there is no need for "reading scores" on the concert platform.

Memory provides our ability to acquire, store, and retrieve information, and my own experiences surprise me. I know I have a current repertoire memory, containing one or two hours of music, but sometimes I can recall and play several minutes of music without any errors, that I last performed twenty or thirty years ago.

This feat of memory surprises me, but it usually happens quite unprompted; I'm simply preparing another piece when a phrase triggers something, and I'm suddenly into the old piece.

So there are definitely long- and short-term memories. I also wonder when I sit at the piano and play, just how it is that my fingers manage to strike the keys so quickly and so accurately.

I have a memory of how to play that seems connected to the music I remember. It all seems automatic. But then I recall where I last played the piece and who was there. So memory has many roles and many different functions.

Memory defined in scientific jargon, is used by the pianist in many ways:

TYPE OF MEMORY [118]	USE BY PIANIST
short term and long term	memorization of scores, short for current repertoire long term for full repertoire
implicit and explicit	explicit for conscious recollection, implicit when using images to remember musical score
declarative	analysis and understand the score
procedural	for remembering keyboard skills and technique
sensory	touché
semantic	expression
episodic	emotional interpretation

I am fascinated by the concept that memory allows me to recall how I felt, that is, exactly what my emotions were in previous times. It seems almost magical, that memories are interconnected, one thought prompting another as vivid as the original event. This happens in our dreams, which are made from the contents of our memory and imagination.[119] Our most strong memories are those that contain emotional and "memorable" events because memory consolidation is effected by the power of the emotional content; big "affects" lead to strong memories.[120]

Quite by accident I learned how to manipulate my musical memory:

Music has always been a visual experience for me, and my earliest and strongest musical memories are of ballet and opera at the Moscow Bolshoi Theatre and, since I started playing piano, I have romanticised and visualised stories to fit my music. This was one of the reasons I was so severely criticised at the Conservatoire for individuality and for moving too much, as I acted my musical stories.

When my MS diagnosis freed me from peer pressure and the straitjacket of classical concerts, it allowed me to indulge and develop my belief in the importance of images to my piano performance.

Just after Hurricane Katrina in the United States I was due to play two Gershwin Preludes in Philadelphia and while learning and rehearsing I visualised images to fit the music. For prelude No 2 C-sharp minor, a television news item of a homeless man plodding through flood water, towing a dinghy holding all of his possessions, including his dog and for prelude No 1 in B-flat, an image of the chaotic Federal Government response by air, rail and road.

These images fitted my interpretation of the music, and for the first time I printed the images and stories in the concert programme. The positive audience reaction ultimately led to creation of video backgrounds that require me to memorise a detailed interpretation of the music, to match the video images.

Using this technique, learning has become quite pleasurable and the process strengthens my memory of the score. This is the same technique used by entertainers who memorise the order of a pack of cards or a long series of numbers. They link the sequence of data to a sequences of images in their personal life, like walking through the parts of their garden or house.

I believe that by consciously creating in memory, a new, visual, emotional "story", based on interpretation of the music, one strengthens and enhances all the memory functions required for performance. There are data supporting the idea that music practice and performance influence the formation of new neurons (adult neurogenesis) in the hippocampus [121] and a lot of data indicating that adult neurogenesis is required for some forms of learning, and of course without learning there is no memory[122].

So my "stories" contain images and feelings from my conscious and possibly subconscious memory. I am not entirely sure if conscious images are essential for feeling emotions, or if emotions automatically lead to conscious images. Possibly emotional feelings can exist and be felt without images, simply in the virtual world of our subconscious.

But what works best for me, is a conscious stream of images, supporting my emotional expression and these possibly stir my subconscious implicit memories.

Ignoring the complexities of creating, editing, and projecting the video, or the restrictions on performance caused by following a visual screenplay, I am absolutely certain that the audience pleasure at these multimedia events is greater than at a formal concert.

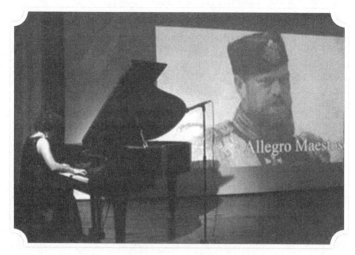

Olga playing a live video concert

I think the images provide a direct route to the subconscious and its distributed cascades of previous memories: sights, sounds, emotions, and so forth. For me this visualisation gives confidence, self-belief, and "reality", making all performance functions more efficient: learning, interpretation, practice and performance itself.

I have discovered that still images are not as effective as moving images; even a simple pan or zoom contributes to the image effectiveness. Presumably our mirror/ motor function needs the stimulation of movement and this leads to the most crucial part of performance technique.

The need for an imaginary narrative to stimulate the associative and cognitive processes that use memory to derive the emotional meaning.

Our imagination drives the associative reward pathway of performance.

CHAPTER 21

Imagine

"Imagine" is a title that was taken by Alan Yentob in his BBC cultural series from the song by John Lennon. For the pianist, however, imagination is the forbidden territory of performance, as the conventional view of "academia" is that musicians convert notes to feelings without any intermediate processes.

But for me this is a false concept that reduces the power of our motor responses and memory and breaks the chain of imagination that connects composer, performer, and audience.

For the listener, imagination commences with an initial limbic valence response that requires identity, a second motor driven valence response of action and intent, both receiving "pleasure" rewards and finally we experience the full emotional meaning of music using our imagination and associative processes.

The functions of the first two stages presumably create the questions of what or who made the sound and what does the sound mean. The answers to these will need the contents of our cognitive brains; they will also need our imagination. To understand what something is or what something means, requires knowledge to provide an explanation. This is supported by research that indicates that sensory and cognitive integration are required to create emotions.[123]

I remember the words of the Simon and Garfunkel hit: "And the vision that was planted in my brain, still remains, within the sound, of silence."[124]

How exactly do we retrieve the visions that are planted in our brain? I have demonstrated to my own satisfaction that memories can be induced or primed by use of images and projected video, but this does not explain the emotional effects of music in the processes of association. Memory formation, location, structure and content in the brain is a complicated and a very active subject in current science. There are learned papers about the importance of the frontal cortex, the amygdala, the medial temporal lobe, the mammillary bodies of the hypothalamus and the hippocampus that connects to the other areas of the cortex, the chemistry and connections of the synapses, and long- and short-term memory effects and plasticity.

One useful fact emerged, which is that exercise seems to enhance memory for both young and old people.[125, 126, 127, 128] This is a good lesson for performers!

Another idea that interested me reading about memory formation was that synapses are emotionally tagged[129] and cross-tagged[130] in some way, involving dopamine. The function that attaches arousal and valence signals to memories provides us with a mechanism for music's influence and impact on our brains.

To reduce this complex subject to performance functions that can be used to enjoy or understand music we need to classify our memories and imaginings for use in performance.

Music is simply a stream of sounds of differing time, pitch, and timbre, but with these attributes I can imagine:

- sounds
- words
- emotions

By visualising and playing "memories" I intend that the audience will sense and appreciate my imaginings.

Sound images are quite simple. For instance, a march requires imagination of soldiers marching; a funeral march requires imagination of a funeral; a waltz requires imagination of dancers waltzing; and a barcarole (gondoliers' song) requires imagination of boats. Beethoven's "Storm Sonata No. 17 in d Minor, Op. 31, No. 2" should conjure up an infinite number of images, including howling wind, lashing rain, rumbling thunder, and strikes of lightning, but none are realised unless you visualise the images.

The challenge for the pianist or indeed any musician is to use real, truthful body language and touché driven by visualized imagery to express music. The secret of generating reality is to link feelings, to the image by remembering specific memories or by creating new ones. For instance, the image of a dancer may become genuinely happy or sad simply by thinking about a happy or a sad dance you have seen or experienced.

Pace and timing have a role to play in our imagination and its connection to our motor responses. Excessive pace reduces the effectiveness of "memory-to-memory" interaction (mirroring).

As our understanding, our basic cognition, is based on what we know, that is, the information in our memory, how can we successfully mirror a dance, a march, or walking at speeds that are not matched in our memory? Imagining a march guarantees the correct speed and my personal taste and the way I teach, requires that music imitates human speeds and rhythms of walking, dancing, marching, and so on. This makes the musical images easier to identify, mirror and enjoy.

One can extend this imitation to other musical phrases and passages representing "audio images", such as the imitation of birdsong and the sound of wind in the branches. By investing reality into the music, one creates intentions that facilitate mirroring. Words, however, do not directly address the mirror functions as their role is higher up the cognitive processes.

CHAPTER 22

Words, words, words[131]

THE CREATION OF visual images in music employs techniques that are used by mime artists who imagine and physically mimic movements without words. However, human civilisation is built on words and languages. Words allow me to quote Aristotle more than 2,000 years after his death or quote Charles Darwin who wrote in 1871:

> "I cannot doubt that language owes its origin to the imitation and modification, aided by signs and gestures, of various natural sounds, the voices of other animals, and man's [sic] own instinctive cries."[132]

I was not really surprised to read that the thesis of Darwin is supported by the findings of the 2007 research of Steeinbels and Koelsch indicating that music and language share similar processes.[133] Their paper investigated semantic and syntactic interactions between music and language in the brain and, very interestingly, indicated that harmonic tension resolution in musical melody is involved in the process.

The evident link between music and language was also described in a fascinating study researching the responses and cry patterns of babies born to groups of French and German mothers.[134] This study showed that babies not only remember music and language but prefer their mother language.

The linguistic preferences shown by the French and German newborns can be partially explained by the physical links between languages and music. These measurable similarities have been demonstrated by Anirudda Patel [135] whose study supports a fascinating theory that music and language share "national characteristics", and these can be analysed through their "Pair-wise Variability Index" (PVI), which measures the patterns of emphasised (long) and non-emphasised (short) syllables or notes.

So the babies respond to linguistic patterns, not words.

This work is spectacularly highlighted by the work of Daniel Everett who spent thirty years studying the Piraha, a small Amazonian tribe whose language,[136] while lacking the concept of numbers, may be sung, spoken, or whistled, thus ensuring that its musical/linguistic PVI is perfectly matched.

There is also a whistled language in the village of Antia on the Greece island of Eubea, and there are drum languages in several parts of Africa. This led to a concept that fascinates me, which is that language can contain meaning that exists independent of words.

Damage to or deterioration of parts of the brain can lead to "aphasia", which is impairment of the ability to recognise or use words. The early work into this condition indicates that damage to Brocas and Wernicke areas of the auditory cortex are responsible for one sub-type of the condition. People who suffer from double aphasia (that is, impairment of recognition and use of words) still try to express themselves with a stream of sound that varies in pitch and pace but has no intelligible words.

There is a fascinating example of this in the book about Tchaikovsky's childhood by his brother Modest, who recalls a story that their cousin Anastasia (their so-called "little sister") expressed herself late in her life, in an unintelligible stream of sounds, presumably because of aphasia associated with dementia.

I have a young piano student with a sibling of two years of age who communicates with his elder sister in an expressive sound stream without recognisable words. She seemingly understands her brother and translates for me when necessary.

So is music a language without words? Yes, most certainly, as more than a hundred, month-old babies exposed to English, nonsense English, English motherese, and unfamiliar languages could discriminate between approval and prohibition in all versions.[137]

They understood the meaning without understanding the words.

We know that language and music are linked by PVI and instinctively we know that music and language are similar, but to unravel the mystery of our understanding of music we need to look in more detail at the things that music and language share.

We all enjoy singing, music with words, and most of us find Rachmaninoff's "Vocalise, Op. 34, No. 14", a song without words, to be enjoyable and moving.

So the irregularly timed patterns that separate the emotional music stream into expressive elements are processed like words. And it appears that this synergy between music and language is a potential benefit for education and for child development.[138] Learning is reinforced by music.

The fact that music may be expressed using linguistic patterns has been instinctive to me, and I use this technique in performance. From my time in the Conservatoire I remember the historical anecdote about Heinrich Neuhaus who used the words "Ām-ster-dam, Ām-ster-dam" to articulate the rhythmic difficulty of phrases in the last movement of Rachmaninoff's "Variations on a Theme of Corelli, Op. 42".

Paul McCartney has told of how he carried a tune around in his head that he called "scrambled eggs" for nearly two years, until he finally wrote the words of "Yesterday".

I regularly "phish" for words, particularly when I need to repeat a musical phrase. I simply fit words to the repetitive phrase, and then by silently repeating the words as I play, I create easy and very subtle variations in expression using the repeated phrase. This prevents mechanical, identical and meaningless repetitions. For instance "open the door, open the door" mimics the beginning of Beethoven's fifth symphony and the repeat of the phrase is never exactly like the first iteration.

It may be that composers do the reverse—they fit music to words as well as words to music.

An example of this may be the main theme of the first movement of Tchaikovsky's "Symphony No. 6 in b Minor, Op. 74, *Pathétique*", something that works in English as well as Russian of me is "May God help me . . . please, may God help me."

But the most complex example "words to music" is the phrase we used to play and at the same time mock, Rimsky-Korsakov and his use of 11/4 time signature in the opera "Sadko". This also works in Russian and English . . . . rim-sky-kor-sa-kov-has-gone-com-plete-ly-mad. You automatically count eleven beats.

Mussorgsky wrote to Rimsky-Korsakov: "Whatever speech I hear, no matter who is speaking . . . my brain immediately sets to working out a musical version of the speech."[139]

In "Promenade" Mussorgsky not only constantly changes rhythm, but he instructs the performer to play "modo russico"—like Russian, he is the master at manipulating complex rhythms.

As a soviet trained musician I feel obliged give the last word to the father of Russian classical musicology, Boris Assafiev about the works of the Godfather of Russian music, Mikhail Glinka in a book that was immediately awarded the Stalin Prize for Literature!

> "the beauty of Glinka lyricism is an automatic unity of tone and word, as such, melody speaks and poetry sings"[140]

The lessons for the pianist is that the brain treats music like language and, therefore, music needs to be played like language, with intent and meaning, in coherent patterns in order to mimic syntax and semantics.

In simple terms the syntax in language is driven by grammatical rules, but there is a natural level of syntax that is above the complication of grammar. It is the syntax of ideas and thoughts governed by relatively simple rules that divides ideas and emotional changes; we call this prosody. This is illustrated by the ability to read out loud. If one is skilled enough and reads slow enough, the brain makes sense before you open your mouth, and the result is coherent and enjoyable. If you read too quickly then the words are simply reproduced as a stream interrupted only by punctuation, the audience has to work hard to find meaning and quickly gets bored by words, words, words.

Forgive me for criticising my idol Tchaikovsky again, but there is a wonderful description of him playing his own composition "Vakula the Smith, Op. 14" to a group of friends only two months before he composed his incredible "Piano Concerto No. 1 in b-flat Minor, Op. 23":

> "Already confused, he "established" himself at the piano and started to play quite badly, not that the whole thing was false or that he stopped at each bar, but in his confusion he was trying too hard, emphasising insignificant elements of the accompaniment and as a result he missed the substance, and the impression was totally unclear. We audience remained silent and the composer, sensing that something was wrong, got even more confused and the whole thing was incoherent, ending up in blushes covered in sweat." [141]

Clearly Tchaikovsky knew the music—he had just composed it, but faced with the score and under pressure, he got lost in the notes and was unable to articulate the sense—the syntax—of the music.

As musicians we must articulate music like speech at a speed the brain can process, If you play too quickly, it is more difficult to articulate the meaning represented by the notes, and if you have to sight read, the problem is infinitely complicated.

The timed electrical activity of the brain can be measured, and science has identified and named "event-related potentials" linked to functional activity. At about 600 milliseconds there is a particular positive electrical peak named P 600. This electrical response is also known as the

Syntactic Positive Shift (SPS), as it relates to the processes associated with syntactic or grammatical error processing.

Other responses like P 400 are also associated with syntactic processing. The knowledge that our brain needs 400-600 milliseconds to commence the process of "syntactic understanding" is hugely important to piano performance.

Music played too quickly increases the risk that "syntactic" mental processing will not convert to "semantic" emotions, regardless of how awesome the speed may be.

Excessive pace will challenge the audience's ability to understand, but it will also make coherent delivery more difficult for the performer. The brain needs to process meaning, so music like language needs expression.

CHAPTER 23

The agony and the ecstasy

I F EXPRESSION IS the key to transmitting emotional meaning with music, how do we, as performers finally unravel the "Gordian knot" of emotion in music, to understand the structure and rules of expression associated with musical melody?

We, as performers, use our instinctive and motor processes to convince the audience to believe and mirror the images and associative emotions that we create from the composer's score, but the final emotional function is not isolated; it is the last of a complex sequence as music passes through the brain.

Before attempting to look at the effects of emotional images, it is worth reviewing the previous chapters and their contributions and inputs to this ultimate function, because we don't consciously feel separate functional effects, we simply listen and experience the music.

The musical brain has a largely sequential architecture with feedback loops that trigger at least three levels of positive and negative reward, involving arousal and valence, the components of emotion.

In the first fractions of a second, the brain processes music tonotopically to assess the pitch height and harmonic quality (timbre) and to make an initial judgement of arousal and valence and possible identity of the source.

The classification of timbre allows individual voices to be separated, and the next process facilitates the establishment of rhythmic patterns and entrainment of voices.

Rhythmic pace combines with pitch height to create a second arousal/valence judgment and rhythmic patterns and time differences, combined with visual signals, also allow the mirror motor responses to make judgements of intent. These include human or non-human actions, possible identity, and some initial meaning.

The audio-processing of harmony has a core function, dividing sounds into octaves and pitch classes to be identified as chroma. A similar function allows the identification of a harmonic progression of fifths that are the basis of the twelve-tone intervals, from which tonality and the scales have been derived for at least 5,000 years.

In addition to the motor images created by pace and rhythms, the brain treats music like language, using word syllabic patterns that require coherent articulation, in order to be associated with specific ideas, motifs, phrases, passages.

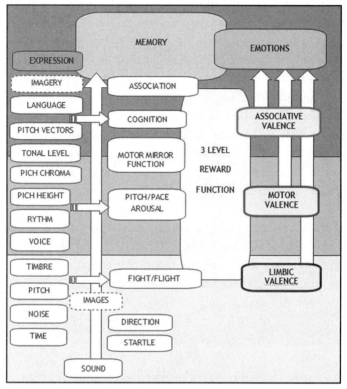

My schema of musical tasks and functions

The diagram of tasks and functions above illustrates my schematic view of the processes.

Finally we come to the interpretation of melody itself (emotional images) for which we already have some clues and indications.

The work of Steeinbels and Koelsch indicates that harmonic tension resolution in musical melody is involved".[142] Musical tension is in fact what we feel as we listen, but instead of the word "tension", perhaps "arousals" is more appropriate.

I already proposed that combinations of pace and pitch intervals can create overall mood or valence for music at the limbic/motor levels, and I am certain that the same relationship is effective in every individual motif, phrase, and passage where the differences in pitch height, up and down and the time difference between successive tones, is the basic generator of arousal and valence, i.e. tension, hence emotions.

Research indicates that the functions that perform the pitch comparison task, involve both halves of the audio cortex.[143] But precisely where in the brain things happen, is less important to me than what is happening.

The concept of pitch vectors in melody also applies to scales which are themselves simple melodies.

It is possible to illustrate the effects vectors by analysis of scales. The diatonic scale is six full tones i.e. two (half-tones) steps that have a constant pitch vector and generate little tension and therefore small resolution when reaching the octave.

Diatonic	T-T-T-T-T-T	or 222222

The basic "chromatic" half-tone scale is even less rewarding than the diatonic scale, as the tone ladder passes octaves without any evident resolution reward.

Chromatic	H-H-H-H-H-H-H etc.	or 11111111 etc.

The Western seven-tone scales has larger tensions and rewards. The major scale contains downward and upward vectors, creating tension and resolution.

Major	T-T-H-T-T-T-H	or 2212221

The minor scales have different, more excessive, downward vector contents.

Natural	T-H-T-T-H-T-T	or 2122122
Harmonic	T-H-T-T-H-TH-H	or 2122131
Rising melodic	T-H-T-T-T-T-H	or 2122221
Descending melodic	T-H-T-T-H-T-T	or 2122122

Strangely enough, different musical scale systems are easily appreciated across cultures. It seems that simply listening is enough to entrain a new scale, what we hear at first may sound strange, but it can quickly become accepted and enjoyed.

The essential part of any sequence of pitch comparison is a starting point, making the key signature the most important attribute of a music. The signature indicates the starting pitch and tonalities (major or minor) of the scale used across the pitch classes.

While I have tried to seek a more empirical method of understanding music, I am left with a caveat—functions are relative, and their effects are subjective and a division of simple pitch height and tonal level are hard to separate. For instance, you will get more response in the higher octaves from a baby; I call this "baby music" when I transpose melodies to octave class six.

This could lead us into stochastic maths to try to define the median pitch level across the population and its relation to perceptions of tonality, but I am happy to accept middle C to be the centre of normal musical arousal, something that then allows me to use the circle of fifths as a basic tonal arousal indicator.

There is also cultural precedence and convention that dictates that certain key signatures reflect certain moods or emotions, which, when defined by the circle of fifths can be understood as arousal steps, marked by sharps and flats.

-6	bbbbbb	$G_b = F_\#$			######	+6
-5	bbbbb	D_b		B	#####	+5
-4	bbbb	A_b		E	####	+4
-3	bbb	E_b	MAJOR	A	###	+3
-2	bb	B_b		D	##	+2
-1	b	F		G	#	+1
0			C			0
			a			
-1	b	d		e	#	+1
-2	bb	g		b	##	+2
-3	bbb	c	MINOR	$f\#$	###	+3
-4	bbbb	f		$c\#$	####	+4
-5	bbbbb	b_b		$g\#$	#####	+5
-6	bbbbbb	$e_b = d\#$			######	+6

Arousal by the circle of fifths

Each progression of the fifths is seven half-tones and this is arousing as a pitch interval, but the arousal of tonal progression is also reinforced by the harmonic relationship first to fifth and the stability of entering a new tonal scale.

This pitch and tonal step can be represented in notation by the number of sharps and flats and these I considered as positive and negative steps of arousal shown on the diagrammatic table.

The table actually represents only part of a spiral, for two reasons: First the steps move between full families of chroma and tonalities that exist throughout the pitch classes of our auditory range.

Secondly +6 and -6, which on the piano, represent the same pitch are ambiguous, furthermore it is possible to increase the number of steps beyond six into a sophisticated world of emotional ambiguity beloved of Chopin.

Even J.S. Bach in his Prelude and Fugue BWV 853 presents us with a dilemma when he writes the Prelude in six flats and the Fugue in six sharps! The two are acoustically identical but they represent emotional opposites.

To illustrate the use of the circle I have a number of other examples; for instance, there is "Ode to Joy" in the key of D major (+2), written by a totally deaf Ludwig van Beethoven as part of the last movement of his "Symphony No. 9". This European anthem demonstrates a positive valence, raises our spirits, unifies our vision, and portrays goodwill.

Other works in this tonality are Pachelbel's canon in D and three famous Violin concertos: Beethoven's "Violin Concerto in D Major, Op. 61", Tchaikovsky's "Violin Concerto in D Major, Op. 35", and Brahms's "Violin Concerto in D Major, Op. 77".

But the work that obsesses the neurological world is a Sonata for two pianos, K. 448, also in D major, which is reputed to generate the magical "Mozart effect"

The first and second movements of Beethoven's "Symphony No. 9" are written in a different tonality, in d minor (-1), which portrays a negative valence: sadness, death, and loss. This is true also of other works: Mozart's "Requiem Mass in d Minor (K. 626)", Max Bruch's "Kol Nidrei, Op. 47", and Haydn's "Missa in Angustiis" ("Mass for Troubled Times"), the mass written for the national memorial service of Lord Nelson.

These works, at the heart of our European musical culture, demonstrate a link between musical tonality and human feelings. D major and d minor appear to be almost opposite emotional worlds. In fact the opposite of -1 is +1 namely G major/e minor, and the best example is Goldberg variations of Bach, for me portraying the entrance to paradise.

Within each musical work the composer moves us up and down emotionally between harmonic sections, by transferring into different tonalities. These steps are relative; there is no book of absolute rules for the starting key signature of works.

Whereas Beethoven is conventional, logical, and systematic, Tchaikovsky is more erratic in his use of tonality, and it seems that each composer has favoured tonalities.

There is a wonderful story in Tchaikovsky's autobiography[144] of how he discovered the trick of transposition, from a young cavalry officer of the Imperial Guard:

> "He told me that he can jump from one tonality to another with just three chords. I was very intrigued and to my amazement I could transport very far, to any tonalities and everything worked."

This event appears to be the point he decided to become a professional musician, because his first surviving composition, "Anastasia Waltz", written before the occasion of the cavalry officer, is in a single tonality.

The same process that generate emotional step or vectors when we move between tonalities, also works at the level of phrases and motifs, where we are moved by pitch steps, up and down, according to scales that are our chosen cultural element of music from which we construct the melodies.

We can think of all music as vectors providing emotional tension giving pleasure when resolved. Clearly rising phrases make positive and happy music, and falling phrases seem sad or negative and this led me to look at the use of rising or falling vectors by different composers.

For example, Beethoven, in his early period, favoured rising phrases, such as in, for example, "Piano Sonata No. 8 in C Minor, Op. 13".

In his later period he was more balanced, but he began to favour falling phrases, for example, in the first movement of "Symphony No. 9 in d Minor, Op. 125".

Tchaikovsky and Chopin are the eternal masters of falling phrases. Just listen to the beginning of the overture to "Eugene Onegin" or "Waltz Op. 69, No. 2".

In his earliest period Mozart was an exponent of rising phrases but this changed later in his life.

Having mentioned Mozart I have to address the "Mozart effect" that fills the Internet with stories of improved spatial reasoning, increased egg yields, the calming of stray dogs and so forth. This magic property of his music is claimed to be so beneficial, it was the subject of some scientific studies[145] by John Hughes who, it appears, successfully achieved reduction in seizure activity of patients in status epilepticus or coma. He stated that periodicity, the repetition of melody and melody reversed, may account for the effect, and in studies of other composers, including J. S. Bach, J. C. Bach, Wagner, Beethoven, Chopin, and Liszt; that Haydn was second to Mozart.

I must say that John Hughes success has not been widely reproduced and for me his analysis of the structure and effects Mozart's music is incomplete.

To explain the wide popularity of Mozart's music both now and in his lifetime, we must start with the fact that he was a child genius writing music from a very young age. This automatically defines his musical style as uncomplicated and simply structured and immature. This is demonstrated by simple consistent rhythms on the beat of the bar, simple voice structures, and the repetitive use of simple melodic phrases. The tonalities of his early works are unambiguously defined by the first and last notes and a predominant use of the first and the fifth notes of the scale throughout the work. This brings a constant confirmation of tonal level by resolution of tensions.

It is evident that this music is easy for the brain to process and success in processing yields constant neural reward, a fundamental reason why many people love Mozart's music but are soon bored by it, like having too much sugar or too many chocolates.

This makes his music both stable and comforting; any collateral effects of listening to his works are based on the fact that the brain is aroused with a positive valence in a stable optimum condition for any other activity.

So the "Mozart effect" for me is a confirmation of my analysis of the functions of music expressed in terms of arousal and valence, driven by changes of pitch, and pace and tension—resolution. If one conducts objective analysis of the these factors one finds that the music of Mozart in not so different to Haydn and other classical period composers and that the earlier baroque works are also similar. These non-romantic works do not require or even allow much expressive input from the pianist.

That does not prevent pianist playing Mozart in a more romantic style, particularly his later works, except that conventional academic education tells us that the composer's score is sacrosanct and that performance must be loyal and accurate to allow members of the audience to interpret the work in their own way. The work of Daniel Levitan at McGill University however tells us the opposite, that expression is the key to enjoyment and for me, expression is the result of interpretation.

My view of interpretation has been criticised by musical neurologist from both east and west, Russia and USA. They fear that a strong interpretation by the pianist, especially using priming images or words, remove from the audience the freedom to create their own interpretation. If this is even partly true, it is an argument for the development of performing computers, not for training physically frail, mentally weak, emotional, memory laden human beings to perform.

With all the priming in the world, every member of the audience is still using their individual memories to understand the interpretation of the pianist. The risk of no expression and no interpretation is that, while the notes alone may stimulate limbic and motor functions they may never trigger associations. For this reason I believe it is necessary to change the view that "notation" defines everything. It doesn't; it provides the structure, the framework, within which the clues to the composer's ideas are encoded.

One can learn to play a score like a computer, without seeking to understand anything, but this results in playing notes without the music. How many times have you listened to your favourite music and suffered agony from an awful performance, when you know that your favourite performer can generate ecstasy?

As artists, we have the final say in vector creation, by our own expression of subtle variations in timing; as we accentuate and clarify the emotions in the music, we create our own agony and ecstasy.

CHAPTER 24

$$E=mc^2$$

T HE CONCEPT OF "time dilation" is an extension of Einstein's theory of relativity, which allows time to be different for observers moving relative to one another, or subject to different gravitational forces.

Four hundred years before Albert Einstein, William Shakespeare wrote, "Time travels in diverse paces with diverse persons."[146]

The idea of time as variable, is a key element of music.

If, like me, you are a YouTube fan, I suggest you view video clips of Chopin's "Étude Op. 10, No. 5, in G Flat Major", as you will find many versions with different tempos. One played by Valentina Lisitsa has had more than 600,000 hits, and there are also versions by Vladimir Horowitz and Lang Lang and some unknown Chinese pianists who are as young as eleven years old.

The speed with which the work is played has driven me to tears of frustration, as I tried to play the tempo defined by my Soviet score, edited by Paderewski and published by the Chopin Institute in 1981, marked Vivace (♩=176), and I have struggled to achieve this published tempo.

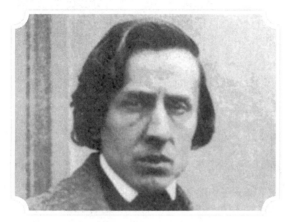

Frederic Chopin

But it took a non-musician just five minutes to tell me that I was a deluded acolyte of the musical cult, loyally believing and following the score.

His argument went like this: Two beats per bar for eighty-four bars is one hundred and sixty-eight beats. At one hundred and seventy-six beats per minute this should take you fifty-seven seconds. At 0.67 seconds per bar, containing six triplets, a strike speed of more than 20 notes per second is required. Impossible.

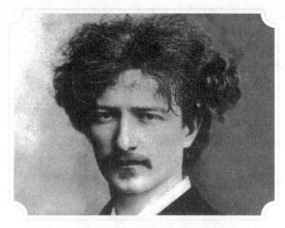

Ignaz Paderewski

You may argue that it is a mistake, a printing error, or that the editor simply did not understand the notation, but reading the accompanying research, it becomes evident that Chopin himself never wrote a single metronome mark on any of the manuscripts. Moreover, the initial French and German published editions contain different tempo instructions.

So if published works can have differences in pace and even permanent errors, it is clear that there can be no such thing as "a correct pace".

To prove this, simply find the YouTube version of this Chopin Étude by Ferruccio Busoni, the Italian, dog-loving, arranger composer friend of my Paul Pabst. Busoni gives the longest performance of all, and even with the noise and poor quality of a 1922 recording it is for me the most musical and the most rewarding.

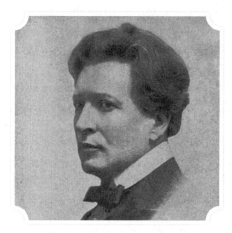

Ferrucio Busoni

The pace of scores without a metronome figure is dictated by the musical notation, which is usually in Italian, for example, Adagio, Alla marcia, Allargando, Allegretto, Allegro, Andante, Largamente, Larghetto, Largo, Lento, L'istesso tempo, Moderato, or Presto, Vivace etc.

While it is possible to find equivalent metronome pace ranges for each term, slavish dedication to pace can be musically destructive; don't be intimidated by the high priests or your peers.

I remember an occasion, rehearsing the Tchaikovsky Trio with a new cellist, when he suddenly stopped and, tapping his bow on the music stand and flourishing his metronome, he said, "This should be 138, and we play only 126."

He had another very strange habit: Every so often he would take a huge noisy breath, which was in no way connected to the music. I can only surmise that his professor had endlessly shouted at him, "Breathe, breathe!" and he simply failed to understand that the music has to breathe and not just chase the metronome.

I have two stories from the past that illustrate pace variability:

The first story concerns Konstantin Igumnov who approached Alexander Goldenweiser after he played Chopin's "Minute Waltz" with the words, "Maestro that was the best five minutes of my life."

Traditionally at the Moscow Conservatoire we were told that Igumnov was mocking Goldenweiser, but knowing their recordings and their long mutual history and that they were both students of Pabst, I understand how much respect Igumnov had for the immense musicality of his friend, and I am more inclined to believe that the remark was a complimentary rather than critical one.

Another story concerns Glen Gould at a recital of a Schubert sonata played by Sviatoslav Richter. Gould is quoted as saying "He started to play as slowly as possible and he took me—time stood still."[147]

Both these pianists were capable of electrifying speed, but both realised that musicality and pleasure are governed by the relationship of pianist to audience, at the time and at the place of performance. Circumstances govern everything: Location, concurrent events, instrument, and the reason for a recital, can all set a mood that dictates the correct tempo; simply remember that Pluchick's field forces affect the person in their environment.

The tempo instructions are simply an indicative frame work into which you fit your interpretation. The process of interpretation never stops and this means that you may never play a piece exactly the same twice.

Time truly does travel at diverse paces in art and in space; E does equal mc^2, it simply depends where you are.

CHAPTER 25

"All the world's a stage"

And all the men and women merely players;
They have their exits and their entrances,
And one man in his time plays many parts.[148]

A S NEUROLOGY AND psychology gradually unravel the secrets of the musical brain, musicians have an opportunity to benefit from new discoveries, to improve their performance capabilities.

By reviewing the "language" of music in the light of current science and elaborating the factors that make music such a powerful medium, we can perhaps explain why so many historic pianists were superstars, whose performances were sublime, but could also be disastrous, and this can help to reverse the decline of the classical genre for the younger generations, giving them the secrets of music and the performing brain, to prepare them to become a new generation of superstars.

In addition to this idealistic educational objective, it is possible that more knowledge of music and brain functions must open up therapeutic and possibly research opportunities.

The first secret of music is self-evident to audiences, but denied by many classical performers:

The musical brain functions on the principle of neural reward that we perceive as pleasure, and therefore music should provide pleasure. To engage the audience, it must entertain.

The performer needs therefore to understand how to stimulate the pleasure mechanisms, that is, how to entertain.

The second secret is that music stimulates the brain's motor processes with minute timing judgements derived from audio and visual signals. These are perceived and interpreted by our mirror function and the performer needs to understand that natural body language is necessary in order to fully engage these neurons.

Performance requires meaningful human actions at the piano, but like magic, it seems sufficient to imagine the actions, to be able to transmit them through touché.

The third secret is that music and language share functions; therefore, music is best expressed like a story, and the performer should understand how to embed and express meanings and feelings in the music, including word images that may already be encoded in the score.

I am convinced that the three secrets need to be used in the process of interpretation to achieve a stage performance. Yes, performing pianists are stage entertainers, regardless of their repertoire.

Finding a meaning for the work establishes the foundation for belief and pleasure to create a spiritual dimension to share with the audience. If there is nothing in your head but stress and a fear of making errors—or a series of notes and notation—the audience will sense that.

Giving pleasure requires that you have pleasure to give. You have to enjoy playing every note of the music.

To use the secrets of meaning and pleasure, you have first to engage the audience, the members of which have arrived for the recital in a multitude of moods (arousals and valances).

Having engaged them, the art of maintaining their interest lies in a continuing dialogue, and this is best achieved by articulating a story.

Capturing the audience requires that they are all entrained to the arousal and valence state of the performer, that is, that they share a similar emotional state or empathy. This is best achieved by directly addressing the audience with a few words, but most performers establish a silence and then use a loud or very soft opening chord. This can gain attention but does not necessarily capture the audience. I find that it is simplest to attempt to entrain the audience at a neutral level, allowing them to share a common mood, typically C major at 65 bpm. It is possible to play a work at a higher pace and slightly more positive valence and achieve a good capture; however, the music must contain a meaning and must be delivered with conviction.

Success is achieved if, at the end of the first piece, audience and performer are sharing an emotional state. Reward comes from performer and audience knowing that they are sharing the same emotions.

Once this level of involvement is achieved, the audience should continue to follow the performer's narrative and feelings, and the programme should have logical connections in order to continue a meaningful dialogue. It is evident that playing all of the waltzes of Chopin in succession, has no entertainment value, and is unlikely to provide sustained pleasure.

As the composer has defined pitch and time signature, the performer is left with the selection of works and the management of pace as the tools to engage, involve, and reward the audience.

In using the word "pace", I mean both the time between and the duration of the notes. I am talking of short and long, fast and slow, acceleration and deceleration, or, in musical terms, tempo, rhythm, rubato, and touché, which are all reflected in our natural body language

False body language and inconsistency between the visual and audio signals, prevents belief and will lose the audience's attention, as the brain processes the timing of body language using both visual and audio information, this is optimised when they are synchronised.

The distance from the piano to the audience should be limited, as the increasing audio delay from the visual image can confuse and detach the two versions of body language, that is, what the audience sees, does not precisely agree with what they hear, if they are too far away.

You may ask what body language is seen when we sit side-on to the audience and look at and strike the keys.

Our body language expresses feelings through our entire being, but the pianist, unlike the actor on stage, remains seated and must allow the precise strike of each key delivering the minute variations of tempo, beat, and touché to become the actions that tell the meaning of the music.

You cannot cheat the mirror neurons, your music must have a meaning.

CHAPTER 26

The secret of my performance triangle

I STARTED THIS NEW book with some simple objectives: to investigate science for musicians and to investigate music for scientists. I also had ambition to substantiate my Triangle of Performance, balancing physical, mental, and emotional functions and capabilities.

The study of the neurology has confirmed and explained many aspects of this—in particular, the differing levels of neurological reward and the function of the motor mirror functions in seeking emotional meaning from physical actions.

Memory, imagination, and belief are crucial to performance. To stimulate them requires a convincing dialogue or story, a technique I have developed during the last four years, through my new "Live Video Music Shows". But I have found that the technique of video in performance is not necessary for achieving a high level of audience pleasure. The key part of the process is the development of the screenplay, the story of the work, the meaning of the music, the question must be: What did the composer mean? Unfortunately this is rarely written in piano scores.

For the singer it is easy—the score has words to explain the meaning of the music. But even for singers, the poetry of the lyrics can be obscure, and then convincing the audience is only achieved if the singer finds and believes in "a meaning"; for example, opera singing in a foreign language can be very unconvincing, something that prevents great Russian operas being popular in the West.

Meaning is simply the conscious or subconscious product of our memory and imagination; composer, pianist, and the audience all imagine a meaning, and it is fairly obvious that if all three agree, the process is likely to be most effective.

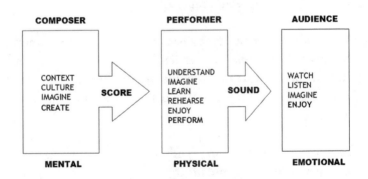

The composer-performer-audience transaction

But if the specific programme was never described by the composer, then it is unlikely that we will discover precisely what he or she meant.

Our objective as performers is to imagine and decide what we think the composer meant. We do this by studying the score, the composer, and the context of the composition.

The meaning may come from the title, the form, and the notation of the work, including the instructions regarding tempo and mood like Affettuoso, Agitato, Animato, Brillante, Bruscamente, Cantabile, Comodo, Con amore, Con fuoco, Con brio, Con Spirito, Con moto, Dolce, Grazioso, Maestoso, Misterioso, Scherzando, Sotto, Semplicemente, or Vivace.

Finally, the use of volume instructions defines the intensity of the mood or tempo, for example, Crescendo, Decrescendo, Diminuendo, Forte, Fortissimo, Mezzo forte, Piano, Pianissimo, or Mezzo piano. Interpretation of these instructions needs to be imagined in the context of the composer, including the times of his or her life and other works.

This background picture allows an interpretation, a meaning to be formulated, understood, and remembered before we play.

For anyone to pretend that it is possible to read and react naturally to these instructions while sight reading, proves that they do not understand the brain processes of arousal and valence.

The display of body language is convincing only if it is natural and subconscious with audio and visual synchronisation. If creating body language becomes part of the conscious processes then our visual actions do not perfectly synchronise with the audio stream, and it is seen as "artificial" and not genuine or "felt".

Real performance can only happen when a work is committed to memory and played freely while imagining the interpretation that we associated with the music.

I have been bitterly disappointed when pianists I considered to be great artists have come to the stage with a score, and you could shut your eyes and listen and know precisely when they turned a page. This never creates great performances.

The interpretation and understanding of a work and the process of turning a sequence of notes into meanings and emotions has to be effected at several levels:

- the whole movement or work
- harmonic sections
- melodic phrases and motifs
- and even individual notes.

In the finest performance every note has a meaning. This requires that the composer intended for every note to have a meaning, and in piano composition only Rachmaninoff and Chopin come close to this perfection.

So the secret of the physical, mental and emotional triangle is: hard work. Learn the score, imagine a meaning, and play every note with conviction.

CHAPTER 27

The triangle of triangles

THE PROCESS OF performing music may be illustrated graphically as a triangle of triangles.

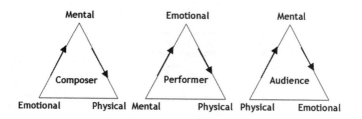

The triangle of triangles

The composer's emotions drive the mental process of composition to create the physical score.

The performer reads the physical score and uses mental capability to generate emotions and create physical sounds.

The audience hears physical sound and uses mental capability to generate emotions.

This simple sequences needs to be expanded in order to fully understand the complexity of the processes and functions involved.

To illustrate this I will describe a typical example.

A composer lives at a time, in a place, within events, with personalities and experiences that are consciously or subconsciously committed to memory.

The act of composing, even if some composers claim that melodies simply come into their heads, cannot be separated from the composer's thoughts and memories. This is the composer's triangle that is shown below.

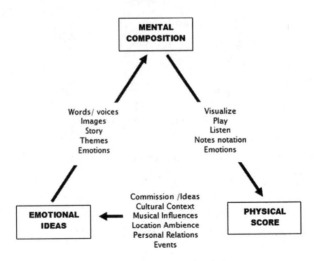

The composer's triangle

Music formulated in the brain uses the composer's "memory", containing his or her cultural environment and his or her emotional state, and therefore these elements are consciously or subconsciously encoded in the composition.

Interpretation of the composition requires creative analysis. As an example I will describe my "interpretation" of "Prelude No. 1 in C Major" from Volume 1 of Bach's "Well-tempered Clavier" BWV 846.

I choose this work for several reasons:

- It is one of the most well-known and popular keyboard pieces of all time.
- There has never been a suggestion that J. S. Bach created this work to any programme.
- It is a work that was written at the time that modern music was defined.

If my claim that the composer's thoughts and memories are subconsciously or consciously encoded into the music is to be shown to be correct, then it must be possible to decode this prelude, which has fascinated me since I first read Albert Schweitzer's classic work on Bach.[149]

Obviously I was not there in 1722 when Bach wrote "Well-tempered Clavier", but I know from the catalogue of his music that Bach was, in keeping with his time, the most prolific composer of religious works. I also know that he wrote two years previously a more simple set of preludes based only on the "white keys" for his son Wilhelm Friedemann Bach.

I believe that in composing the "Well-tempered Clavier" Bach was, for the first time, trying to define the "musical universe" of the full keyboard and, by inference, "God's musical universe".

Where does one start in defining "God's musical universe"? Simply, "In the beginning"—the first phrase in the book of Genesis.

So I concluded that the story of the creation—"the beginning"—might be coded into Bach's first prelude.

In solving the secret of the composer's triangle, I read, understood, and created a story that I could believe.

My preparation for performance is represented by the second triangle, that requires analysis of the score, marking the significant harmonic changes, which indicate the composer's ideas developing, like scene changes in a film. The analysis identifies the arousal value of each tonal section on a scale of +6 to -6, equivalent to the position on the circle of fifths, or the sharps and flats of the key signature.

I was not surprised to find that "Prelude No. 1 in C Major" from Volume 1, has seven harmonic changes, which might depict the seven days of creation. Coincidence? Does it matter? No. I believe I found a sense in the work that allows me to empathise with the composer.

Having imagined a meaning and fixed the scene changes, I can analyse the tempo, the rising or falling phrase patterns, and vectors. Then, together with the scales, harmony, tension, and resolution, I evolve the screenplay.

This analysis of the score is not an academic exercise; it is an exciting forensic investigation that supports both the playing and learning of a work, serving to develop increasing empathy with the composer and define meaning for the movements, passages, phrases, and motifs.

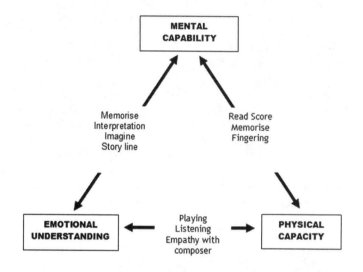

The performer's learning triangle

The process is greatly assisted by the evolution of visual images for the storyline that unite the score, the sound of music to my physical movements.

The learning process is more efficient and enjoyable when the notes in the score are enhanced in memory by visual images and emotions.

I had "divine" assistance interpreting the first prelude. The analysis of the musical score used the words of the bible. NB In the baroque period, works do not contain large shifts in tonality.

BAR 1-4 C major 0	And the earth was without form, and void; and darkness
First day. BAR 5-11 to G major +1	And God called the light Day, and the darkness he called Night
Second day BAR 12-15 unresolved C major -1 to 0	Let there be a firmament in the midst of the waters, And God called the firmament Heaven
Third day BAR 16-19 confirmed C major O (one class lower)	God called the dry land Earth; and the gathering together of the waters called he Seas: and God saw that it was good. Let the earth bring forth grass, and the fruit tree yielding fruit God saw that it was good.
Fourth day BAR 20-24 unconfirmed F major -1	And God made two great lights; the greater light to rule the day, and the lesser light to rule the night: he made the stars also.
Fifth day BAR 25-28 unconfirmed C major O	God created great whales, and every living creature that moveth, which the waters brought forth abundantly, after their kind, and every winged fowl after his kind:
Sixth day BAR 29-32 dominant of C major with dissonances	And God made the beast of the earth, and cattle and every thing that creepeth upon the earth and Made man in his image, to have dominion over all
Seventh day BAR 33-35 fundamental of C major	He sanctified it: because that in it he had rested from all his work

As the practice/rehearsal proceeds, the ideas, words, images, score, and notes modify and strengthen the memories of musical audio and my finger sequences. Performance becomes an enjoyable replay of the memorised musical story.

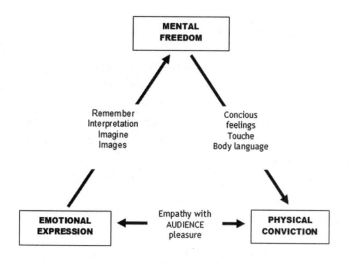

The performer's stage triangle

On the stage, I simply remember the story elements and visualise images, and then the recall of music requires little mental effort: It is pleasurable and easier than reading a score.

This technique is explained by Eckhart Altenmuller's research showing that, if it carries a valence, music can evoke strong emotions in an audience that can be remembered for years. Strong emotions seem to facilitate memory formation and retrieval.[150]

This research works for the performer as well as the audience, but the performer has a much greater need for memory enhancement than an audience. The concert pianist has to remember thousands of physical note sequences, their notations, and the melodies they create.

The collateral benefits of my method of associating stories and images with music, are:

- I do not feel alone on the concert platform.
- The score has been replaced by a musical story that is robust in memory and is easy to recall.
- By imagining, I experience emotions, and these are manifested in genuine and believable body language.
- The process gives me pleasure that the members of the audience can share.

Finally, the Audience Triangle: The audience hears the music, watches the performer, and empathises. However, without some priming or previous memory of the music this may be difficult to achieve. When primed the audience will begin to imagine and link music to their own memories, ideally with the performer's body language being part of the process.

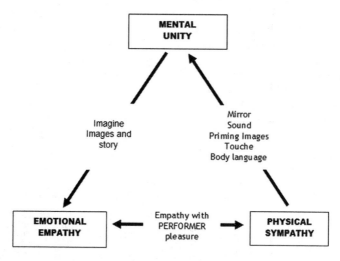

The audience triangle

To achieve maximum audience participation, the performer has to understand that:

- Music is a language.
- Music is written with the intention of imparting ideas, emotions, and images.
- Its interpretation and understanding are based on memories and emotions.
- Appreciation is based on pleasure (neurological rewards in the brain), shared by the performer and audience.
- Pace and rhythm must match brain-processing speeds and mirror human motion and natural images.
- Increasing tone, pace, and volume creates arousal and valences
- Key signatures and tonal changes in the score represent emotional valence variations.

- Naturally expressed variations of these parameters, maintain the audience's attention and belief.
- One has to believe to be believed.

The different styles of music, such as baroque, classical, romantic, and impressionist, have different notations and features that become evident in the analysis.

As we progress towards the peak of the romantic genre, emotions are more accentuated, and the music contains more imagery. In Beethoven we imagine trees, mountains, storms, dances, and so on, and we feel pain, sadness, triumph, and so forth. In his "Symphony No. 5 in C Minor", the opening—"Da Da Da Dam, Da Da Da Dam"—in his own words, according to Anton Schindler, his secretary and biographer, is, "Thus, fate knocks at the door."[151]

When arranging passages of Vivaldi "Four Seasons" at the request of a "mature" student who wanted to play her favourite music. I was astonished to find, in the early baroque score, realistic physical instruction intended to evoke the imagination of the performers derived from a sonnet, here is the verse about winter[152]:

Allegro non molto

Aggiacciato tremar trà nevi algenti	To tremble from cold in the icy snow,
Al Severo Spirar d' orrido Vento,	In the harsh breath of a horrid wind;
Correr battendo i piedi ogni momento;	To run, stamping one's feet every moment,
E pel Soverchio gel batter i denti;	Our teeth chattering in the extreme cold

Largo

Passar al foco i di quieti e
contenti
Mentre la pioggia fuor bagna
ben cento

Before the fire to pass peaceful,
Contented days while the rain
outside pours down.

Allegro

Caminar Sopra il giaccio, e à
passo lento
Per timor di cader girsene
intenti;
Gir forte Sdruzziolar, cader à
terra
Di nuove ir Sopra 'l giaccio e
correr forte
Sin ch' il giaccio si rompe, e si
disserra;
Sentir uscir dalle ferrate porte
Sirocco, Borea, e tutti i Venti in
guerra
Quest' é 'l verno, mà tal, che
gioja apporte.

We tread the icy path slowly and
cautiously,
for fear of tripping and falling.
Then turn abruptly, slip, crash
on the ground and, rising,
hasten on across the ice lest it
cracks up.
We feel the chill north winds
course through the home
despite the locked and bolted
doors . . .
this is winter, which nonetheless
brings its own delights.

So if images are good enough for Vivaldi . . . What more do I need to say?

As with any human communication, the secret of efficient transmission of meaning is based not on the content but in maintaining belief and interest by variation of tone, timbre and valence, rhythm and pace, and so on.

As music is the unique art form in which interpretation by a performer is required, it is essential for the performer to understand not only the physical score but the mental creativity and emotional intentions of the composer and also the probable effects of the music on the audience.

If a performer plays an unconvincing interpretation, one can be prompted to leave a concert of even of a favourite work. I have done so on more than one occasion, from some very expensive seats.

This proves to me that the notes themselves are not the music. The music is the sympathetic human interpretation that completes the empathy trail from composer via the performer to the audience, a spiritual transaction with a wonderful mystery:

How does sad music gives as much pleasure as happy music?

CHAPTER 28

Brain restoration

T HINKING ABOUT THE mystery of how sad music can give pleasure, I found myself reflecting on my own experiences and why I can truthfully say that MS changed my life for the better.

You may wonder how, after a diagnosis of multiple sclerosis, I can be so optimistic about the future. The reasons are very simple: MS forced me to look at my life and my music with a new focus, creating new directions and targets.

The limitations of MS forced me to look at music, not as I had previously, as a frustrating and often unrewarding performance career; I stopped chasing recording contracts and professional engagements, as my diagnosis simply made them unrealistic.

My first lifeline was teaching and the increasing rewards that come with experience and with feedback from students, many of whom are now dispersed around the world in the United States, China, Japan, Germany, Estonia, and France.

The second lifeline was research into my country's musical history, and the novel that grew out of the characters I studied.

A third lifeline—analysing performance—grew out of the first two, by helping my students learn from the lessons of history and from neurological knowledge that evolved from my research.

But all of this was made possible by my MS treatments, which have given me both confidence and expectation of new therapies and have blurred my first horrific thoughts of a musical demise like Jackie Du Pré.

So instead of struggling with one life, I now enjoy four. I still play for MS and record DVDs of most of the concerts. I teach. I research and I write.

As for neurology and music, this book is simply the beginning. I intend to spread my ideas as widely as possible in the musical and neurological worlds, and I relish the prospect of defending my unconventional ideas.

My continuing work in the MS world constantly reminds me that there are many worse off than me, and some of the most badly challenged, live very positive and fulfilled lives that inspire me.

Forgive me for all of the stories of the Silver Period and my musical heroes in a book that is intended as a serious analysis of performance and the brain, but we only make sense of things with the content of our own brains.

Each time I enter my lounge and touch my beautiful Schroeder, I have the feeling that my brain has been restored, like my piano. I insisted that the ivory keys should be untouched so that my direct connection with their past would remain unbroken.

I dream that maybe at least one of my musical heroes played my piano, alas not Tchaikovsky, as the piano was built two years after his death.

But the G3 ivory keeps coming loose, and this I think is the voice of the maestro Tchaikovsky in his favourite tonality, telling me to get on with my story about him. I have new information and a closeness to his history that comes from ten years of research, travelling to the places he visited, standing on the ground he walked, and reading the letters that he wrote.

One particularly poignant discovery was the French estate of his friend and benefactress Nadezhda Von Meck.

I finally traced her Chateau Belair near Tours in 2010 and walking by the carp lake, the little handkerchief-sized fields, and the quiet alley of trees that she described to him in her letters, I mused how different things may have been if he had taken her invitation to visit her French "Pleschéevo" and play the Erard she had bought for him.

The one thing that was not mentioned in her letters was the discretely placed little cottage in the grounds of the chateau that she may have intended as his private workspace.

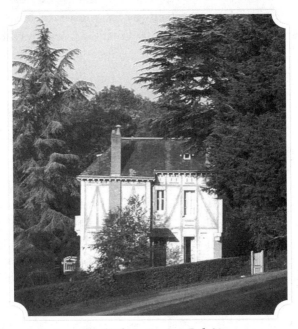

The little cottage at Belair

After Tchaikovsky's refusal to visit, Nadezhda sold the chateau at a large loss and just four years later they were both dead, he burdened by debt and she alone, in Nice on the French Rivera where the manuscripts of history tell us that Nadezhda died with a painful neurological condition in Villa Skariatine, which was fitted with a cold bath treatment room and stood opposite the clinic of Dr Donaudy, an acolyte of Dr Charcot who first identified multiple sclerosis and cold water treatments. I speculate she may have had MS.

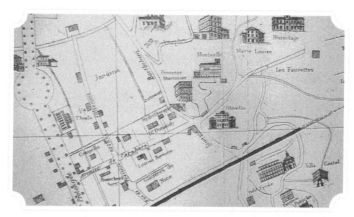

Nadezhda Von Meck's last home in Nice: Villa Skariatine

But even stranger: Belair near Tours is now the Croix-Rouge National Neurological Rehabilitation Centre of France.

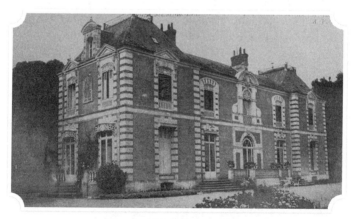

Von Meck's Belair c. 1900

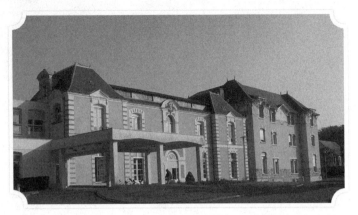

National Red Cross Neurological Centre in Belair

When I visited Belair and played in the sports hall for the patients, I was simply devastated to have four members of the audience flat in bed in a vegetative state. One in particular made me cry; he was a handsome young pilot who lay lifeless, and I have no way of knowing if the music had any benefit for him.

But I am convinced we need to research harder, in a more focused and empirical way, to discover the secrets of music and the brain.

ABOUT THE AUTHOR

O LGA BOBROVNIKOVA IS a Moscow Conservatoire-
trained concert pianist with multiple sclerosis (MS).
This disease could have destroyed her life and career;
instead, it changed her life. Dedicating her career to MS
under the symbolic Mu-Sic title. She taught, researched,
and wrote about Russian musical history and questioning
the decline of pleasure in modern piano performance
Olga decided to unravel the secrets of pleasure and the
performing brain.

ABOUT THE BOOK

B EING CONSTANTLY CRITICISED for excessive emotion and movement by her piano professors, Olga Bobrovnikova took inspiration and a new attitude to performance when she heard the recordings made in the 1890s of a forgotten pianist, Paul Pabst, who Tchaikovsky has called "a pianist blessed by God".

Her diagnosis of MS coincided with her discovery of Pabst and his music, and in her typically defiant way, she set out to record Pabst's exceptionally difficult piano paraphrases of Tchaikovsky operas as well as a trio that has been dedicated to Anton Rubinstein and also to make the first ever recording of Pabst's own piano concerto.

Her research into Pabst was like a backdoor into the secrets of Russian musical history, which led to Olga's novel *The Diaries of Alexandra Petrovna*. She was drawn by the circumstances and their relationship to the conclusion that Pabst's was the hidden hand that Tchaikovsky admitted he needed to help with the passages of his "Piano Concerto No. 1".

Her immersion in this lost history of the Russian Piano School revealed major differences in and controversy regarding the style of piano performance as well as coinciding with a growing interest in the brain and music. A passion for pleasure in performance and a study of the neurology of her MS-damaged brain created this unique book, which is a fusion of fascinating musical history, a wide review of scientific research, and detail of a new performance method.

Professor Cyril Hoschl: "The book is really impressive!"

Professor Gavin Giovannoni: "A very interesting read"

Professor Andrew Lees: "Outrageous comments are what is needed in a sea of ignorance."

Professor Jean-Pierre Malkowski: "A fascinating story and account of your life experiences."

Professor Blanka Schaumann: "An eye-opening approach to understanding of the relationship between music and the brain . . . . [T]his is truly original and it will open new pathways."

Professor Lawrence S Sherman ". . . . the book is very interesting and there are some great threads that run through the book. I feel that it has the seeds to be a truly great and unique contribution".

Prof Jŭrg Kesserling ". . . congratulations on your interesting and well written book!"

ENDNOTES

1   Correspondence between Professor Lawrence Sherman and
     Olga Bobrovnikova

2   Correspondence between Tchaikovsky and Von Meck

3   *The Dawn of Recording* (Marston Records).

4   Norman Lebrecht, *When the Music Stops . . . : Managers,
     Maestros and the Corporate Murder of Classical Music*
     (London: Simon & Schuster, 1996).

5   Olga Bobrovnikova, *Paraphrases on Themes By
     Tchaikovsky—Pabst, P.* Talent Records Oct 2003

6   Julius Block, *Life under Three Tzars* (unpublished)

7   *Freddie Mercury: The Great Pretender* (Director's Cut) (Eagle
     Roc Productions, 2012).

8   Salmon VN, Benovoy M, Larcher K, Dagher A, Zatorre RJ
     Anatomically distinct dopamine release during anticipation
     and experience of peak emotion to music.

9   Professor Richard Muscat, Associate Professor Physiology
     and Biochemistry, Faculty of Biomedical Sciences and
     Surgery, Pro-Rector for Research and Innovation, The
     University of Malta.

10   "Arthur Rubinstein Obituary", *The New York Times*, 21
     December 1982.

11   Anne J, Blood, and Robert J. Zatorre, "Intensely Pleasurable
     Responses to Music Correlate with Activity in Brain Regions
     Implicated in Reward and Emotion".

12   S. L. Bengtsson, and F. Ullén, "Dissociation between Melodic
     and Rhythmic Processing during Piano Performance from
     Musical Scores".

13   Quotation is attributed to Hans Von Bülow.

14   Olga Bobrovnikova, *Triangle of Performance* (2006).

15   Society for Neuroscience, <www.sfn.org>.

16   M. P. Mattson, W. Duan, and Z. Guo, "Meal Size and Frequency Affect Neuronal Plasticity and Vulnerability to Disease: Cellular and Molecular Mechanisms".

17   Glenn Doman, and Janet Doman, *How Smart is Your Baby?* (New York: Square One Publishers, 2006).

18   Trevor W. Robbins, and Barry J. Event, "Neurobehavioural Mechanisms of Reward and Motivation".

19   Carlos Juri, MariCruz Rodriguez-Oroz, and Jose A. Obeso, "The Pathophysiological Basis of Sensory Disturbances in Parkinson's Disease".

20   Smith KS, Berridge KC, Aldridge JW. "Disentangling pleasure from incentive salience and learning signals in brain reward circuitry".

21   Cited in Helmholtz (1954), p. 251.

22   T. Fritz et al., "Universal Recognition of Three Basic Emotions in Music".

23   B. H. Pierce, and E. A. Kensinger, "Effects of Emotion on Associative Recognition: Valence and Retention Interval Matter".

24   Carolina Labbé, and Didier Grandjean, "Rhythm, Entrainment and Musical Emotions".

25   Marcel Zentner, et al., "Emotions Evoked by the Sound of Music: Characterization, Classification, and Measurement".

26   Johann Mattheson, *Das Neu-Eröffnete Orchester* (Hamburg: B. Schiller, 1713), pp. 161 and 167; Beekman C. Cannon, *Johann Mattheson: Spectator in Music* (London: Yale University Press, 1947), p. 129.

27   Jonna K. Vuoskoski, and Tuomas Eerola, "Measuring Music-induced Emotion Models, Personality Biases, and Intensity of Experiences".

28 C. Sansone, Carolyn C. Morf, and A. T. Panter (eds), *The SAGE Handbook of Methods in Social Psychology* (: SAGE Publications, 2003).

29 Jack et al., Dynamic Facial Expressions of Emotion Transmit an Evolving Hierarchy of Signals over Time, Current Biology (2014), http://dx.doi.org/10.1016/j.cub.2013.11.064

30 Berridge KC, Robinson TE, Aldridge JW. "Dissecting components of reward: 'liking', 'wanting', and learning".

31 William Forde Thompson, *"Exploring Variants of Amusia: Tone Deafness, Rhythm Impairment, and Intonation Insensitivity"*.

32 S. E., Trehub, T. Vongpaisal, and T. Nakata, *"Music in the Lives of Deaf Children with Cochlear Implants"*.

33 T. Hopyan, K. A. Gordon, and B. C. Papsin, *"Identifying Emotions in Music through Electrical Hearing in Deaf Children Using Cochlear Implants"*.

34 C. J. Limb, *"Cochlear Implant-mediated Perception of Music"*.

35 J. K. Chen, et al., "Music Training Improves Pitch Perception in Prelingually Defined Children with Cochlear Implants".

36 Hyde KL, Zatorre RJ, Griffiths TD, Lerch JP, Peretz I. "Morphometry of the amusic brain: a two-site study".

37 Will U. Bigan, et al., "The Time Course of Emotional Responses to Music".

38 Suzanne Filipic, Barbara Tillmann, and Emmanuel Bigand, "Judging Familiarity and Emotion from Very Brief Musical Excerpts".

39 M. Roy, et al., "Modulation of the Startle Reflex by Pleasant and Unpleasant Music".

40 J. F. Schouten, "The Perception of Timbre", in Y. Kohasi (ed.), *Reports of the 6th International Congress on Acoustics, Tokyo, GP-6-2*, 6 vols (Tokyo: Maruzen, 1968), 35-44.

41 Jaeho Seol, et al., "Discrimination of Timbre in Early Auditory Responses of the Human Brain".

42   James W. Lewis, et al., "Human Cortical Organization for Processing Vocalizations Indicates Representation of Harmonic Structure as a Signal Attribute".

43   Will U. Bigan, et al., "The Time Course of Emotional Responses to Music".

44   C. D. Tsang, and N. J. Conrad, "Does the Message Matter? The Effect of Song Type on Infants' Pitch Preferences for Lullabies and Playsongs".

45   Dorothy Bruck, Ian Thomas, and Vincent Rouillard, "How Does the Pitch and Pattern of a Signal Affect Auditory Arousal Thresholds?", *Journal of Sleep Research*, 18/2 (2009), 196-203.

46   L. Lanteaume, et al., "Emotion Induction after Direct Intracerebral Stimulations of Human Amygdala".

47   B. H. Pierce, and E. A. Kensinger, "Effects of Emotion on Associative Recognition: Valence and Retention Interval Matter".

48   Jaeho Seol, et al., "Discrimination of Timbre in Early Auditory Responses of the Human Brain".

49   James W. Lewis, et al., "Human Cortical Organization for Processing Vocalizations Indicates Representation of Harmonic Structure as a Signal Attribute".

50   Séverine Samson, Robert J. Zatorre, and James O. Ramsay, "Deficits of Musical Timbre Perception after Unilateral Temporal Lobe Lesion Revealed with Multidimensional Sealing".

51   Chakalov I, Draganova R, Wollbrink A, Preissl H, Pantev C. Oct 2013"Perceptual organization of auditory streaming-task relies on neural entrainment of the stimulus-presentation rate: MEG evidence".

52   M. Pressman, *Little Corner of Musical Moscow in the 1880s: In the Memory of Professor* (Moscow: State Publisher, 1962).

53   Published by Carl Fischer in Boston, Massachusetts in 1892.

54 Letter from Ferruccio Busoni to Gerda Sjöstrand, 27 January-8 February 1895, Mosca.

55 Solo of "Ballade pour Adeline", *BBC Breakfast*, February 2013.

56 I. Szirmai, "How Does the Brain Create Rhythms?".

57 Chen J. L., Penjune V. B., Zatorre R. J. (2008). Listening to musical rhythms recruits motor regions of the brain.

58 Hui-Min Wang, "A Pysiological Valence/Arousal Model from Musical Rhythm to Heart Rhythm".

59 L. Bernardi, C. Porta, and P. Sleight, "Cardiovascular, Cerebrovascular, and Respiratory Changes Induced by Different Types of Music in Musicians and Non-musicians: The Importance of Silence".

60 J. C. Shaw and K. R. McLachlan, "The Association between Alpha Rhythm Propagation Time and Level of Arousal".

61 Dorita S. Berger, "Pilot Study Investigating the Efficacy of Tempo-specific Rhythm Interventions in Music-based Treatment Addressing Hyper-arousal, Anxiety, System Pacing, and Redirection of Fight-or-Flight Fear Behaviours in Children with Autism Spectrum Disorder (ASD)".

62 J. S. Snyder, and E. W. Large, "Gamma-band Activity Reflects the Metric Structure of Rhythmic Tone Sequences".

63 U. W. Weger, et al., "Things are Sounding Up: Affective Influences on Auditory Tone Perception".

64 Annie Lang, Kulijinder Dhillon, and Oingwen Dong, "The Effects of Emotional Arousal and Valence on Television Viewers' Cognitive Capacity and Memory", Journal of Broadcasting & Electronic Media, 39/3 (1995).

65 See Chapter 6

66 G. Musacchia, E. Large, and C. E. Schroeder, "Thalamocortical Mechanisms for Integrating Musical Tone and Rhythm".

[67] E. O., Flores-Gutierrez, et al., "Metabolic and Electric Brain Patterns during Pleasant and Unpleasant Emotions Induced by Music Masterpieces".

[68] D. Deutsch, "The Octave Illusion in Relation to Handedness and Familial Handedness Background", *Neuropsychologia*, (1983).

[69] Diana Deutsch, Trevor Henthorn, and Rachael Lapidis, "Illusory Transformation from Speech to Song".

[70] J. D. Warren, et al., "Separating Pitch Chroma and Pitch Height in Human Brain".

[71] Manuel S. Malmierca, et al., "A Discontinuous Tonotopic Organization in the Inferior Colliculus of the Rat".

[72] Lakshmi Chandrasekaran, Ying Xiao, and Shobhana Sivaramakrishnan, "Functional Architecture of the Inferior Colliculus Revealed with Voltage-sensitive Dyes".

[73] Titze, I.R. (1994). Principles of Voice Production,

[74] Baken, R. J. (1987). Clinical Measurement of Speech and Voice.

[75] "Neurology", Charlie Rose, Bloomberg TV, 2011.

[76] Bruce Eldine Morton, "Left-brain, Right-brain Differences between Opponents at Sites of Recurring Aggression: Discovery of Familial Polarity, a Biological Factor tied to Conflict".

[77] Letter No.

[78] T. K. Perrachione, et al., "Evidence for Shared Cognitive Processing of Pitch in Music and Language".

[79] Postscript of Jurgenson's letter to Tchaikovsky, 1 January 1878, OS.

[80] Catherine Drinker Brown, *Free Artist: The Story of Anton and Nicholas Rubinstein* (: Little, Brown & Co., 1939), p. 270.

[81] Kwang-chich Chang, et al., *The Formation of Chinese Civilization: An Archaeological Perspective* (Beijing: Yale New World Press, 2005).

[82] "Joanna Lumley's Greek Odyssey", Tiger Aspect Productions Ltd for ITV, 2011.

[83] Andrew Barker (ed.), *Greek Musical Writings*, 2 vols (Cambridge, UK & New York: Cambridge University Press, 1984-9)

[84] H. G. Wells, *The Outline of History* (New York: The Macmillan Company, 1921), p. 258.

[85] "Power of Pentatonic Scale—Demonstration by Bobby McFerrin", YouTube, at the event "Notes Neurons: In Search of the Common Chorus" from the 2009 World Science Festival.

[86] Tillmann B Implicit investigations of tonal knowledge in non-musician listeners.

[87] Janata P. Brain networks that track musical structure.

[88] Petr Janata, et al., "The Cortcal Topography of Tonal Structures Underlying Western Music".

[89] J. D. Warren, et al., "Separating Pitch Chroma and Pitch Height in the Human Brain".

[90] Rizzo M, Eslinger PJ. Colored hearing synesthesia: an investigation of neural factors.

[91] Sir Isaac Newton, *Opticks: or, A Treatise of the Reflections, Refractions, Inflections and Colours of Light.*

[92] Seth Pancoast, *Blue and Red Light; or, Light and Its Rays as Medicine* (1877).

[93] Edwin D Babbett, *The Principles of Light and Color* (1878).

[94] Oscar Von Riesman, *Recollections of Rachmanioff.*

[95] Ronald McGregor, et al., "Function of Diurnal Phase, Operant Reinforcement versus Operant Avoidance and Light Level".

[96] G. Svaetichin, "Spectral Response Curves from Single Cones" (1956).

[97] Aristotle cited in Helmholtz (1954), p. 251.

[98] Istvan Molnar-Szakacs and Katie Overy, "Music and Mirror Neurons: From Motion to 'E' Motion".

[99] Stefan Koelsch, "A Neuroscientific Perspective on Music Therapy".

[100] M. Roy, et al., "Modulation of the Startle Reflex by Pleasant and Unpleasant Music".

[101] S. Koelsch, T. Fritz, and G. Schlaug, "Amygdala Activity Can Be Modulated By Unexpected Chord Functions during Music Listening".

[102] Chia-Jung Tsay, "Sight over Sound in the Judgment of Music Performance".

[103] J. Van den Stock, et al., "Instrumental Music Influences Recognition of Emotional Body Language".
J. Van den Stock, et al., "Instrumental Music Influences Re

[104] Randolph Blake and Maggie Shiffrar, "Perception of Human Motion".

[105] N. Logeswaran and J. Bhattacharya, "Crossmodal Transfer of Emotion by Music".

[106] M. A. Meredith and B. E. Stein, "Visual, Auditory, and Somatosensory Convergence on Cells in Superior Colliculus Results in Multisensory Integration".

[107] K. Alaerts, S. P. Swinnen, and N. Wenderoth, "Interaction of Sound and Sight during Action Perception: Evidence for Shared Modality-dependent Action Representations".

[108] E. Ricciardi, et al., "Do We Really Need Vision? How Blind People 'See' the Actions of Others".

[109] Istvan Molnar-Szakacs and Katie Overy, "Music and Mirror Neurons: From Motion to 'E' Motion".

[110] Dezhe Z. Jin, Naotaka Fujii, and Ann M. Graybiel, "Neural Representation of Time in Cortico-basal Ganglia Circuits".

[111] J. A. Grahn, "The Role of the Basal Ganglia in Beat Perception: Neuroimaging and Neuropsychological Investigations", *Ann N Y Acad Sci*, 1,169 (2009), 35-45.

[112] P. Loui, et al., "A Generalized Mechanism for Perception of Pitch Patterns".

[113] Aurélie Bidet-Caulet, et al. "Listening to a Walking Human Activates the Temporal Biological Motion Area".

[114] Stephen M. Rao, Andrew R. Mayer, and Deborah L. Harrington, "The Evolution of Brain Activation during Temporal Processing".

[115] Carlos Juri, MariCruz Rodriquez-Oroz, and Jose A. Obesoa, "The Pathopysciological Basis of Sensory Disturbances in Parkinson's Disease".

[116] F. T. Van Vugt, H. Jabusch, and E. Altenmüller, "Individuality That is Unheard of: Systematic Temporal Deviations in Scale Playing Leave an Inaudible Pianistic Fingerprint".

[117] Anjali Bhatara, et al., "Perception of Emotional Expression in Musical Performance".

[118] P. Fietta and P. Fietta, "The Neurobiology of the Human Memory".

[119] Bradley R. Buchsbaum, et al., "The Neural Basis of Vivid Memory is Patterned on Perception".

[120] Iván Izquierdo, et al., "Different Molecular Cascades in Different Sites of the Brain Control Memory Consolidation".

[121] Wei Deng, James B. Aimone, and Fred H. Gage New neurons and new memories: how does adult hippocampal neurogenesis affect learning and memory?

[122] Prof Larry Sherman in e-mail to Olga Bobrovnikova

[123] E. O. Flores-Gutierrez, et al., "Metabolic and Electric Brain Patterns during Pleasant and Unpleasant Emotions Induced by Music Masterpieces".

[124] Paul Simon and Art Garfunkel, "The Sound of Silence, 1964.

[125] M. G. Dik, et al., "Early Life Physical Activity and Cognition at Old Age" (2003).

[126] C. H. Hillman, K. I. Erickson, and A. F. Kramer, "Be Smart, Exercise Your Heart: Exercise Effects on Brain and Cognition" (2008).

[127] J. R. Nocera, et al., "Can Exercise Improve Language and Cognition in Parkinson's Diseases?" (2010).

[128] L. Chaddock, et al., "Aerobic Fitness and Executive Control of Relational Memory in Preadolescent Children" (2011).

[129] S. Sajikumar and J. U. Frey, "Late-associativity, Synaptic Tagging, and the Role of Dopamine during LTP and LTD".

[130] S. Frey and J. U. Frey, "'Synaptic Tagging' and 'Cross-tagging' and Related Associative Reinforcement Processes of Functional Plasticity as the Cellular Basis for Memory Formation".

[131] William Shakespeare, *Hamlet*, Act 2, Scene III.

[132] Charles Darwin, *The Descent of Man, and Selection in Relation to Sex* (1871).

[133] N. Steinbeis and S. Koelsch, "Neurocognition of Music".

[134] B. Mampe, et al., "Newborns' Cry Melody is Shaped by Their Native Language".

[135] A. D. Patel, et al., "Processing Syntactic Relations in Language and Music: An Event-related Potential Study".

[136] Daniel L. Everett, *Don't Sleep There are Snakes* (2008).

[137] Anne Fernald, "Approval and Disapproval: Infant Responsiveness to Vocal Affect in Familiar and Unfamiliar Languages".

[138] S. Moreno, et al., "Musical Training Influences Linguistic Abilities in 8-year-old Children: More Evidence for Brain Plasticity".

[139] Diana Deutsch, "Speaking in Tones: Music and Language Partner in the Brain".

[140] Boris Asafiev, Academician "M. I. Glinka" 1947 U. S. S. R. State publishing house,

[141] N. Kaskin, *Memoirs of P. I. Tchaikovsky* (Moscow, 1896), p. 92. [Published in Russian.]

[142] N. Steinbeis and S. Koelsch, "Neurocognition of Music".

[143] N. Angenstein and A. Brechmann, "Left Auditory Cortex Involved in Pairwise Comparisons of the Direction of Frequency Modulated Tones".

[144] Cited by Kashkin in *Memoirs of Tchaikovsky* (Moscow: 1896).

[145] John R Hughes, "The Mozart Effect: Additional Data", *Epilepsy Behav*, 2 (2001), 369-417.

[146] William Shakespeare, *As You Like It*, Act 3, Scene II.

[147] William Shakespeare, *As You Like It*, Act 2, Scene VII.

[148] *The Enigma*, dir. Sviatoslav Richter (, 1998). [Documentary about Bruno Monsaingeon.]

[149] Albert Schweitzer, *Johan Sabastien Bach* (Music Publishing, 1965 [1904]). (in Russian)

[150] S. Eshrich, T. F. Munte, and E. O. Altenmüller, "Unforgettable Film Music: The Role of Emotion in Episodic Long-term Memory for Music".

[151] Anton Schindler, *Life of Beethoven*, ed. Ignace Moscheles (London: Henry Colburn, 1841).

[152] Wikipedia